Institute of Pathology, Laboratory and Fo

Universiti Teknologi MAR

PURE TOCOTRIENOLS AND TOCOTRIENOL-TOCOPHEROL MIXED FRACTION AS ANTI-ATHEROSCLEROTIC AGENTS

SUHAILA ABD MUID
GABRIELE RUTH ANISAH FROEMMING
ABDUL MANAF ALI
HAPIZAH MD NAWAWI

Research Book

Institut Patologi, Perubatan Makmal Dan Forensik (I-PPerForM)
Faculty of Medicine, Universiti Teknologi MARA,
Sg Buloh Campus, 48000 Sg Buloh, Selangor,
Malaysia.

ISBN: 9781792721625

First Published: December 2018

Amazon Kindle Direct Publishing

ABSTRACT

Tocotrienols (TCTs) is a more potent antioxidant than tocopherol (TOC). However, the role of Tocotrienol enriched mixed fraction (TEMF) and pure TCT isomers as a potential potent anti-atherosclerotic agent in human ECs compared to pure α-TOC is not well established. The anti-atherosclerotic mechanism of TCTs is also unclear. The objectives of this study were to investigate (i) the effects of TEMF, pure TCT isomers, and α-TOC on inflammation, endothelial activation, monocytes binding activity, NFκB and eNOS, and (ii) the most potent pure TCT isomers on the inhibition of the inflammation, endothelial activation, monocytes binding activity, NFκB and eNOS biomarkers in lipopolysaccharides (LPS) stimulated human ECs. Human umbilical vein endothelial cells (HUVECs) were incubated with various concentrations of TEMF, pure TCT isomers and α-TOC (0.3-10 µM) together with, lipopolysaccharides (LPS) for 16 hours. Culture medium and cells were collected and measured for the protein and gene expression of cytokines, adhesion molecules, NFκB and eNOS. Delta (δ)-TCT is the most potent TCT isomers in terms of as an atheroprotective agent. TEMF and pure TCT isomers exhibit anti-atherosclerotic properties with great potential as atheroprotective agents. The possible pathway for its anti-atherosclerotic activity is through the NFκB deactivation. α-TOC has inhibitory effects on the anti-atherosclerotic properties of TCTs in TEMF.

TABLE OF CONTENTS

Contents

5

CHAPTER ONE
INTRODUCTION

1.1 BACKGROUND AND PROBLEM STATEMENTS

Atherosclerosis is a slowly progressing disease of the medium and large sized arteries and characterized by formation of fatty and fibrous lesions in the vessel wall (Winther et al., 2005). As a result, it will lead to serious atherosclerosis-related clinical complications such as stroke, peripheral vascular diseases (PVD) and cardiovascular diseases (CVD) (Hanssons & Hermansson, 2011). To date, CVD remains the major cause of mortality in the world, typically claiming a third of all deaths (Lonn et al., 2011). Inflammation and endothelial activation are the early stages in the development of atherosclerosis. During these stages, there will be over expression of cytokines [Interleukin-6 (IL-6)] and adhesion molecules [intercellular cell adhesion molecule-1 (ICAM-1), vascular cell adhesion molecule-1 (VCAM-1) and e-selectin] by the ECs (ECs) (Leeuw et al., 2005). Therefore, it is suggested that IL-6, ICAM-1, VCAM-1 and e-selectin can be used as useful predictive biomarkers towards atherosclerotic progression and new targets of treatment (Poredos, 2011).

ECs are sensitive to oxidative stress and gravity alterations (Buravkova et al., 2005). ECs produce active molecules such as cytokines [IL-6 and tumor necrosis factor-alpha (TNF-α)], ICAM-1, VCAM-1 and e-selectin in response to injury or oxidant stimuli (Osiecki, 2004). Increasing numbers of these active molecules will facilitate the transmigration of monocytes into the tunica intima, the key step in the initiation of atherosclerosis.

Epidemiological studies have indicated the beneficial effects of Vitamin E in reduction of cardiovascular events but in various clinical trials, the results were contradictory (Rimm et al., 1993; Stampfer et al., 1993; Brigelius-Floh, 2007). In a meta-analysis report, high dosage of Vitamin E in humans (> 150 IU/day or 100 mg/day) increased all causes mortality and should be avoided (Miller et al., 2005). However, such conclusions may not be appropriate when only α- Tocopherol was tested in that meta-analysis (Gee, 2011). In addition, α-Tocopherol is often incorrectly referred to as vitamin E. Vitamin E actually consists of both tocopherols and tocotrienols. The existence of tocotrienols is almost always disregarded in vitamin E research (Khanna et al., 2005).

Tocopherols (TOCs) and tocotrienols (TCTs) are collectively called tocols (Khosla et al., 2006). They are composed of a chromanol ring with an attached phytyl side chain. Both tocols consist of four isomers (α-, β-, γ- and δ-) according to the presence of methyl groups and all of them are active vitamers of vitamin E (Nakagawa et al., 2007). TCTs differ from TOCs by possessing three double bonds in the phytyl side chain (Baliarsingh et al., 2005). High concentrations of TCTs are present in crude palm oil and extracts from the fruits of *Elaeis guineensis* (Maclellan, 1983). The advantages of palm oil derived TCTs when compared to TOCs is that it has more potent anti-oxidant, anti-cancer, anti-aging, anti-thrombotic and anti-angiogenic activities (Sen et al., 2007). However the information on TCTs as an anti-inflammatory and anti-endothelial activation agent especially in ECs is still lacking. Even though several reports on the inhibitory effects of TCTs on endothelial activation have been reported previously, further investigation is warranted especially on the pure TCT isomers (Theriault et al., 2002; Naito et al., 2005). The link between endothelial nitric oxide synthase (eNOS) and nuclear factor kappa B (NFκB) mediated pathways leading to the reduction of cytokines and adhesion molecules is need to be investigated. In addition, inhibition of monocytes binding activity to ECs by TCTs is not well established. It has been suggested that any intervention that can finally lead to the inhibition of monocyte binding activity is the best target adjuvant or supplementation in slowing down the progression of atherosclerosis. This is base on the fact that, the initiation of monocytes into the tunica intima through the transendothelial migration process cells is the key event to the pathogenesis of atherosclerosis (Cook-Mills & McCary, 2010).

1.2 SCOPE OF STUDY

The potential use of tocotrienol-enriched mixed fraction (TEMF) and TCT isomers (α-, β-, γ- and δ-) in the reduction of protein and gene expression of inflammation and endothelial activation and eNOS upregulation in LPS stimulated EC was determined. Furthermore, the pathway potentially involved in the reduction on those biomarkers through NFκB deactivation was also being studied. In addition, the most potent pure TCT isomers that give beneficial effects in the reduction /induction of the above mention biomarkers were determined in this study.

1.3 OBJECTIVES

General objectives: To study the effects of TEMF, pure TCT isomers and α-TOC on inflammation and endothelial activation in stimulated ECs: Protein and gene expressions analysis and the possible pathway.

The specific objectives:

a) To investigate the effects of TEMF on protein and gene expression of inflammation and endothelial activation, monocytes binding activity, NFκB and eNOS.

b) To determine the effects of pure TCT isomers and α-TOC on the inhibition of these above mention biomarkers in stimulated EC.

c) To determine the most potent TCT isomers on the reduction of protein and gene expressions of inflammation, endothelial activation, monocytes binding activity, NFκB and eNOS.

1.4 HYPOTHESES

a) TEMF reduces protein and gene expression of inflammation and endothelial activation, monocytes binding activity, NFκB and increases eNOS.

b) Pure TCT isomers and not α-TOC reduces protein and gene expression of inflammation and endothelial activation, monocytes binding activity, NFκB and increases eNOS.

CHAPTER TWO
LITERATURE REVIEW

2.1 ENDOTHELIAL CELLS

The entire vascular endothelium in the blood vessels is built up from endothelial cell (ECs) monolayers (Sumpio et al., 2002). In an adult, the endothelium consists of approximately 1×10^{13} of ECs (Sumpio et al., 2002). Figure 2.1 illustrates the scanning electron microscopy picture of a blood vessel with the ECs lining.

The origin of ECs during embryogenesis is under debate (Munoz-Chapuli et al., 2005). However, it has been suggested that ECs and hematopoietic cells (HPC) share the same precursor cells, the hemangioblast which originates from the mesoderm mainly in the areas closer to the endoderm and also in the aorta–gonad–mesonephros region (Sumpio et al., 2002). The hemangioblast will then transform into intermediate pre-ECs and differentiate into either a committed HPC cells line or ECs (Sumpio et al., 2002).

In contrast to human fibroblast and smooth muscle cells, ECs grew as homogenous monolayers of large polygonal cells and centrally located nucleus (Jaffe et al., 1973). Weibel-Palade bodies (rod-shaped cytoplasmic organelle) are the special characteristic of ECs that cannot be seen in other cell types i.e. smooth muscle cells and fibroblast. In addition, ECs contain abundant quantities of smooth muscle actomyosin and major blood group antigens (ABH) (Jaffe et al., 1973).

The vascular endothelium is an active metabolic component of tissues. It serves several important physiological functions such as regulation of microvascular fluid and solute exchange, maintenance of anti-thrombogenic vessel surface, modulation of vascular tone and blood flow and regulation of immune and inflammatory responses by controlling monocytes interaction with the vessel wall (Kvietys & Granger, 1997). ECs allow for a fine regulation of blood flow through the production of nitric oxide (NO) by the endothelial isoform of the nitric oxide synthase or eNOS (Munoz-Chapuli et al., 2005).

FIGURE 2.1

Scanning Electron Microscopy Picture of a Blood Vessel With ECs Lining
Source: Steve Gschmeissner, Photo Researchers Inc (2009)

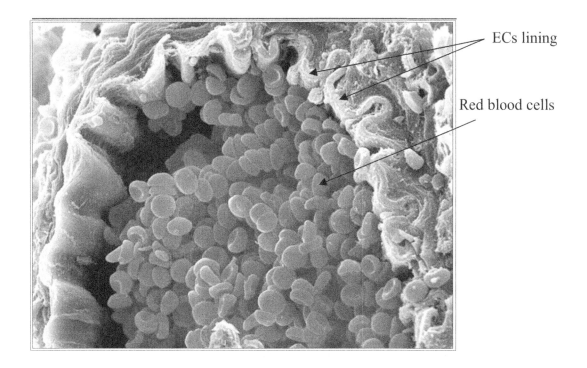

ECs lining

Red blood cells

Various functions of ECs are illustrated in Figure 2.2. Abnormal endothelial cell response has been associated with organ dysfunction and disease; this has led to an intense interest in developing an *in vitro* model system to study endothelial cell dysfunction i.e. inflammation and endothelial activation (Kvietys and Granger, 1997).

The most common approach for isolation of endothelial cells is from the internal lining of large blood vessels, such as human umbilical veins endothelial cells (HUVECs) (Feairheller et al., 2011). HUVECs have been recommended as an *in vitro* model to investigate inflammatory and endothelial activation processes in atherosclerosis because it has been suggested that HUVECs responses to any stimuli closely mimic those responses of true *in vivo* endothelial cells (Onat et al., 2011).

Eventhough the usages of human artery endothelial cells (HAECs) as an *in vitro* model for atherosclerosis study are increasing, the usage of HUVECs are still relevant. It is due to the current report by a group of investigator showing that the upregulation of chemokines, adhesion molecules and enzymes involved in inflammation in response to TNF-α by HUVECs was comparable to HAECs (Jefferson et al., 2013). Previous investigators has also reported that venous EC have a similar capacity to arterial EC to release vasoactive factors, thus supporting the hypothesis that veins have a functional endothelium that may modulate venous tone (D'Orleans et al., 1992). In addition, HUVECs and HAECs have similar properties by carrying oxygenated blood in humans.

FIGURE 2.2

Various Function Of ECs
Source: Poredos (2011)

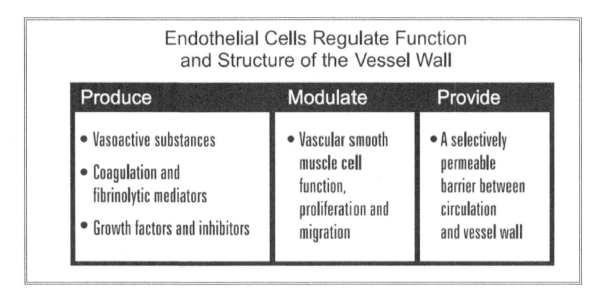

ECs can be activated in response to various stimuli such as wounds, infections and presence of cytokines, after which there will be an alteration of their functions (Grosse et al., 2012). As a defence against infection and unintentional blood clotting, ECs will transmit signals to vascular smooth muscle, thrombocytes and other cells (Pearson, 2000). Stimulation of ECs with lipopolysaccharides (LPS) has been shown to enhance the production of IL-6 and adhesion molecules such as ICAM-1, VCAM-1 and e-selectin (Lim et al., 1998). It has been reported that the basal level of expression and kinetics of LPS stimulated expression of ICAM-1 on HUVECs are qualitatively similar to observation in various tissues of rats (Panes et al., 1995). Production of cytokines and adhesion molecules can be further detected by sensitive enzyme linked immunoassay (ELISA) method in conditioned media obtained from cell culture (Constans & Conri, 2006).

2.2 INFLAMMATION

Inflammation is a necessary part of the immune response where it represents a highly co-ordinated set of events that allow tissues to respond against injury or infection (Babu et al., 2009). Acute inflammation is initiated through the production of cytokines (i.e. IL-6 and TNF-α), resulting in the delivery of leukocytes to the site of injury or infection (Fergusona, 2010).

However chronic inflammation may occur when the inflammatory process persists or sustains over a period of time (Fergusona, 2010). Among the causes of chronic inflammation are prolonged chemical exposure, persistent foreign bodies and recurrent acute inflammation (Talwar et al., 2011). Increased risk of chronic disease may occur as a result of chronic inflammation (Fergusona, 2010). Atherosclerosis is the result of chronic inflammation where previously, it has been considered to be mainly a disorder of lipid metabolism (Sata & Fukuda, 2011). It is generally accepted that vascular areas of atherosclerotic progression are in a state of persistent inflammation (Scrivo et al., 2011). As a consequence, any further inflammatory stimulus in the sub-intimal area automatically becomes a proatherogenic stimulus and altering the behaviour of the intrinsic cells of the artery wall. Then, recruitment of inflammatory cells will further promote lesion formation and complications (Leonarduzzi et al., 2012). The interest in predictive markers of inflammation in cardiovascular disease has increased because it has been proven that inflammation initiates and maintains the formation of atheromatous plaques in coronary and peripheral arteries (Francisco et al., 2006). It has been shown that inflammation led to increase expression of cytokines and adhesion molecules in both *in vitro* and *in vivo* studies (Packard & Libby, 2008).

LPS stimulates immune cells/ECs to trigger the inflammatory response though activation of various pathways (i.e. NFκB activation or STAT-3). This response is characterized by the release of an array of pro-inflammatory mediators, IL-6 which results in a signal transduction of numerous pro-inflammatory genes (Martinez et al., 2012). Transcription factors such as NFκB or STAT-3 is transactivated when pro-inflammatory cytokines (TNF-α or IL-6) ligate their receptors on the endothelial surface (Wung et al., 2005). In response to that, sICAM-1, sVCAM-1, e-selectin and p-selectin are leukocyte adhesion molecules that are rapidly synthesized by ECs to facilitate monocyte recruitment into the vessel wall across an intact endothelium, a key event in the pathogenesis of atherosclerosis (Hansson, 2001).

In terms of inflammation and atherosclerosis, IL-6 and TNF-α are suggested as the useful biomarkers (Poredos, 2011). Biomarkers can consist of any entity that occurs in the body that can be measured to predict the diagnosis, onset or progression of a disease process (Maiese et al., 2010).

2.2.1   Interleukin-6

IL-6 is the pleoitropic cytokine with a wide range of biological activities such as immune regulation, hematopoiesis and cell proliferation (Naka et al., 2002). IL-6 receptors can be found on normal resting T-cells, myeloid cells, activated normal B-cells, keratinocytes, mesengial cells and ECs (Willerson & Ridker, 2004). In normal function, IL-6 is involved in cells differentiation of osteoclasts and megakaryocytes and immunoglobulin production by B-cells (Naka et al., 2002).

IL-6 is also the main cytokine with a broad range of humoral and cellular immune effects relating to inflammation, host defense and tissue injury (McCarty, 1999). IL-6 release from activated ECs triggers synthesis of acute-phase proteins [C-Reactive Protein (CRP)] in the liver via binding to IL-6 receptors on hepatocytes (Heinrich et al., 2003). When IL-6 is released into the systemic circulation, the endothelium increases the release of adhesion molecules and plasma concentrations of fibrinogen and plasminogen activator inhibitor type 2 (PAI-1) which amplifies inflammatory and pro-coagulant responses (Paoletti et al., 2004). IL-6 is the main pro-atherogenic cytokine and has a strong association with atherosclerosis (Thusen et al., 2003). IL-6 is produced and secreted by ECs, smooth muscles cells as well as macrophages (Yudkin et al., 2000).

Several investigators have reported that serum levels of IL-6 are elevated in hypercholesterolaemic patients, and were positively correlated with the level of oxidized LDL (ox-LDL) (Harris et al., 1999). It has been shown that IL-6 gene transcript is expressed in human atherosclerotic lesions as well as in genetically hyperlipidaemic rabbits (Seino et al., 1994; Ikeda et al., 1992). In a prospective clinical study conducted among post-menopausal women, IL-6 was associated with the increased risk of cardiovascular events, although it was not an independent predictor after adjustment in a multivariate model (Ridker et al., 2000). Patients with unstable angina were reported to have elevated IL-6 levels which is associated with poor outcomes (Yamashita et al., 2003). Therefore, it has been suggested that reduction of IL-6 by therapeutic interventions could be cardioprotective and gives better outcome among patients with high risk of getting CAD (Swerdlow, 2012).

2.2.2 Tumor Necrosis Factor-Alpha

Tumor necrosis factor-alpha (TNF-α) is a pleiotropic inflammatory cytokine which belongs to the TNF superfamily (Zhang et al., 2009). In normal body regulation, low levels of TNF-α is important in maintaining homeostasis by regulating body circadian rhythm and promotes the remodeling or replacement of injured and senescent tissue by stimulating fibroblast growth (Tracey & Cerami, 1990).

TNF-α is a key mediator in the local inflammatory immune response which is implicated in the pathogenesis of atherosclerosis (Zhang & Zhang 2011). TNF-α is produced by several cells involved in the atherosclerotic process including ECs, macrophages, lymphocytes and smooth muscle cells (Blake & Ridker, 2002). TNF-α levels elevation in humans are reported in advanced heart failure and associated with increased risk of recurrent coronary events (Hegewisch et al., 1990).

In atherosclerosis, TNF-α activates NFκB via a canonical/classical pathway to induce the expression of adhesion molecules (Orange et al., 2005). ECs upon stimulation by TNF-α produce e-selectin, and subsequently macrophages and ECs produce ICAM-1 to promote the macrophages accumulation in tunica intima (Blake & Ridker, 2002). TNF-α regulates NOS expression and/or activity, which exerts direct effects on NO production (MacNaul & Hutchinson 1993). TNF-α decreases eNOS expression in ECs and diminishes NO production leading to endothelial dysfunction (Zhang et al., 1997; Goodwin et al., 2007). It has been reported that intra-arterial TNF-α infusion in human provides direct evidence about TNF-α stimulated vascular dysfunction (Chia et al., 2003).

2.3   ENDOTHELIAL ACTIVATION

Endothelial activation is an immunological and inflammatory response that promotes the secretion of adhesion molecules, induction of pro-coagulant molecules and elicitation of T-cell mediated immune responses (Zhang et al., 2010). ECs activation is responsible for the formation of the atherosclerotic plaque and vascular wall inflammation, a major contributor to atherosclerosis (Altman, 2004). Figure 2.3 shows that the endothelial activation leads to a cascade of events in the formation of atherosclerotic plaque.

There are two types of endothelial activation processes. Type I EC activation occurs immediately following stimulation and does not require de novo protein synthesis or gene transcription. Type II EC activation is a delayed response for several hours or days that is independent on the activation of gene transcription and the de novo synthesis of proteins (Zhang et al., 2010).

During Type I EC activation, ECs release restored protein such as p-selectin, thrombin and histamine before the endothelium in the venules and small veins rapidly retracts and leading to hemorrhage, edema and increases vascular permeability (Bach et al., 1994).

During Type II EC activation, there is an upregulation of adhesion molecules (ICAM-1, VCAM-1), cytokines (IL-6 and TNF-α), chemokines and pro-coagulant genes (Cines et al., 1998). It has been reported that during this initial stage, endothelium expressed e-selectin on its surface and releases Von Willebrand Factor (VWF), interleukin-8 (IL-8) and platelet-activating factor (PAF) (Hunt & Jurd, 1998).

FIGURE 2.3

**ECs Activation Leads to Cascade Of Events In The Formation Of Atherosclerotic
Plaque
Source: Pradhan & Sumpio (2004)**

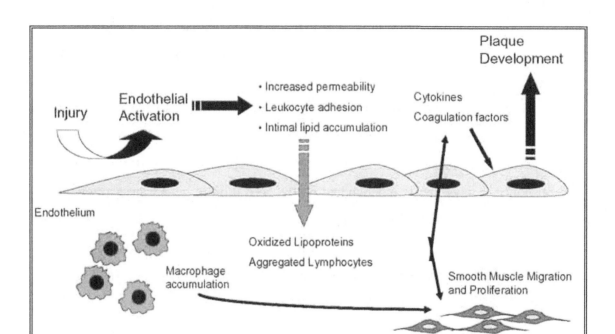

Ultrastructural alterations of the ECs have been observed during Type II EC activation and it is characterized by protrusion of ECs into the lumens of blood vessels, hypertrophy of ECs, increase in biosynthetic organelles (Golgi complex, rough endoplasmic reticulum and ribosomes), increase in permeability and appearance of monocytes and lymphocytes in the vicinity of activated ECs (Lawson & Wolf, 2009).

ECs activation represents a reversible endothelial alteration resulting in morphological rearrangement (increase in cell size and cytoplasmic organelles) and inducible new functions but without loss of endothelial integrity (Cotran, 1989). Type I and Type II ECs activation is reversible upon the withdrawal of EC activators (cytokines, TNF-α, and interferon) (Pober, 1998). Uncontrolled activation processes can progress to ECs apoptosis which represents irreversible endothelial injury, endothelial fragmentation and EC separation from intima (Zhang et al., 2010). EC activation may also lead to endothelial dysfunction, the imbalance between relaxing and contracting factors (NO and endothelin) (De Meyer & Herman 1997). In addition, endothelial dysfunction involves disruption of its vasoactive role in regulating tissue perfusion (Szmitko et al., 2003) and may play an important role in the development and maintenance of high blood pressure (Hedner et al., 2000). Endothelial dysfunction with irreversible EC injury can be produced by uncontrolled chronic and persistent ECs activation over months (Zhang et al., 2010). Persistent EC activation can result in critical local levels of endothelial adhesion molecule (ICAM-1, VCAM-1, e-selectin) cytokines (IL-6), pro-coagulant molecules, vasodilators and chemokines (Zhang et al., 2010). IL-6, ICAM-1, VCAM-1, and e-selectin have been recommended as surrogate biomarkers of endothelial activation (Zhang et al., 2010). Soluble forms of ICAM-1, VCAM-1 and e-selectin are present in the supernatant of cytokine-activated ECs after 18 hours of incubation period (Pigott et al., 1992). It has been suggested that biomarkers of ECs activation can also serve as sentinels for ECs injury/damage or endothelial dysfunction (Zhang et al., 2010).

2.3.1 Intercellular Cell Adhesion Molecules-1

Intercellular cell adhesion molecule-1 (ICAM-1) (CD54) is another member of the immunoglobulin-like cell adhesion molecules expressed on many cell types such as ECs, smooth muscle cells and monocytes (Lawson & Wolf, 2009). ICAM-1 is involved in the trans-endothelial migration of leukocytes to sites of inflammation (Lawson & Wolf, 2009). The interaction of leukocytes integrins [leukocytes function-associated antigen-1 (LFA-1) and macrophage 1 antigen (Mac-1)] with ICAM-1 permits the adhesion and transmigration of leukocytes through the endothelium (Tsakadze et al., 2002). ICAM-1 can be induced in ECs through a cytokine dependent pathway, bacterial LPS and oxygen radicals (Tsakadze et al., 2002). ICAM-1 expression is upregulated in arterial ECs at lesion areas in hypercholesterolaemic mice and rabbits (Liyama et al., 1999). The presences of ICAM-1 in these atherosclerotic lesions are associated with the progression of atherosclerosis (Lawson & Wolf, 2009).

Soluble form of ICAM-1 is detectable in the blood and other body fluids (Tsakadze et al., 2002). There is a significant association between increase sICAM-1 concentrations and future CAD in healthy individuals (Wallen et al., 1999). Diabetes mellitus, obesity, low high-density lipoprotein levels (HDL-c) and hypercholesterolaemia increases the plasma sICAM-1 levels in blood (Bermudez et al., 2002; Ito et al., 2002). It was suggested that among healthy subjects, sICAM-1 concentrations predict the risk of acute myocardial infarction and diabetes mellitus (Ridker et al., 1998). Furthermore, it has been suggested that, circulating sICAM-1 is a marker of ICAM-1 activation on ECs (Mills et al., 2002). The exact mechanism by which sICAM-1 is expressed has not been yet identified (Lawson & Wolf, 2009). However, it has been postulated that the presence of sICAM-1 soluble expression in plasma is due to the enzymatic cleavage of cell surface ICAM-1 (Champagne et al., 1998; Tsakadze et al., 2004). Among the proposed candidate proteases are matrix metalloproteinases (MMP), human leukocyte elastase and TNF-α -converting enzyme (TACE) (Lyons & Benveniste, 1998; Sultan et al., 2004). Other possible pathways are the activation of TNF-α, interleukin-1β (IL-1β) and interferon-γ through the mitogen-activated protein kinase (MAPK), Src thyrosine kinase and Phosphatidylinositol 3-kinases (PI3K) pathway which induce sICAM-1 to be shed off from the cell surface of various primary cells and cell lines (Lawson & Wolf, 2009).

Beside its role in leukocyte emigration, ICAM-1 also transmits intracellular signals leading to the rearrangement of the actin cytoskeleton and activation of pro-inflammatory cascades that can be responsible for an inflammatory response (Lawson & Wolf, 2009).

2.3.2 Vascular Cell Adhesion Molecules-1

Vascular cell adhesion molecule-1 (VCAM-1) or CD106 is a member of the immunoglobulin-like adhesion molecules expressed on activated ECs (Ley & Yuqing, 2001). VCAM-1 is primarily involved in mediating both rolling-type adhesion and firm adhesion of monocytes and lymphocytes to the endothelium via integrin $\alpha_4\beta_1$ (Chen et al., 1999). In comparison with ICAM-1, VCAM-1 pattern regulation is unique because it is not expressed under baseline condition (Ley & Yuqing, 2001). VCAM-1 is rapidly induced by the inflammatory cytokine TNF-α, LPS, interleukin-1 (IL-1), IL-6 and its induction is sustained for 48 to 72 hours.

VCAM-1 can also be induced by lysophosphatidycholine and other oxidized phospholipids in ECs (Kume et al., 1992). Such phospholipids species are generated during lipoprotein oxidation and this may explain the increased adhesive properties of ECs exposed to ox-LDL. VCAM-1 is also induced by pro-atherosclerotic conditions in rabbits, mice and human including in early lesions (Hilis, 2003).

There was evidence of VCAM-1 expression on the luminal aortic endothelium (Li et al., 1993). VCAM-1 expression was induced in aortic endothelium of rabbits as early as seven days after initiation of an atherogenic diet (Li et al., 1993). VCAM-1 has also been observed in areas of neovascularization and inflammatory infiltrates at the base of plaques, suggesting that intimal neovascularization may be an important site of inflammatory cell recruitment into advanced coronary lesions (Cockerill et al., 1995). In addition, sVCAM-1 was proposed to be correlated with risk of developing acute coronary syndrome in patients with established cardiovascular disease (Guray et al., 2004). Findings from several investigators have suggested the involvement of VCAM-1 in neointima formation because it facilitates monocytes infiltration into injured arteries (Manka et al., 1999).

2.3.3 E-Selectin

E-selectin, a member of the selectin family molecules, is an endothelial-specific adhesion molecule and specifically expressed on the surface of stimulated ECs (Kansas, 1996; Eppihimer et al., 1996). It has been reported that E-selectin induced by cytokines is expressed on the ECs of venules and capillaries, but not the EC of arterioles or arteries (Pober & Cotran, 1990). In addition, E-selectin is expressed on the EC of medium or small size veins but not the EC of the aorta (Fries et al., 1993). Soluble e-selectin may be released by enzymatic cleavage or may result from damaged or activated ECs (Vestweber & Blanks, 1999). In addition, soluble e-selectin concentrations appear to correlate with its expression on the surface of HUVECs (Leeuwenberg et al., 1992). E-selectin has been suggested as a marker of endothelial activation. E-selectin consists of an amino terminal "C type" lectin domain critical for ligand interaction, an epidermal growth factor-like domain, six complement regulatory repeats, a single transmembrane domain and a cytoplasmic carboxyl-terminal tail (Yu et al., 2004). E-selectin is important for the adhesion of polymorphonuclear leucocytes, monocytes and lymphocytes in cytokine-stimulated HUVECs (Bevilacqua et al., 1989). It mediates slow rolling and stable arrest of monocytes on the endothelium during inflammation (Kunkel & Ley, 1996; Milestone et al., 1998). It also enhances the subsequent recruitment of monocytes by capturing them from the axial stream, and enable them to roll along the endothelium (Wood et al., 2006).

The role of e-selectin in cardiovascular disease has been extensively reviewed (Roldan et al., 2003). E-selectin levels are increased in patients with unstable angina or myocardial infarction compared to normal controls (Blann et al., 1996). In addition, a high level of e-selectin is found in patients with hypercholesterolaemia, low high density lipoprotein (HDL-c), obesity, hypertension and diabetes mellitus (Constans & Conri, 2006).

2.4   MONOCYTE - ECs BINDING

The adherence of monocytes to the vascular endothelium and subsequent migration of cells into the vessel wall are an important early event in atherogenesis. Monocytes adherence to ECs is mediated by cell adhesion molecules such as ICAM-1, VCAM-1 and e-selectin (Vasanthi et al., 2012). Pro-inflammatory cytokines such as IL-6 induces ECs to release chemotactic factors and cell adhesion molecules and subsequently contributes to the inflammatory process (Ludwig et al., 2004).

Adhesion molecules and chemokines are the most important mediator of mononuclear cell adhesion to the arterial wall, as its cognate ligand, the integrin very late antigen-4 (VLA4) is selectively expressed on monocytes (and some T-lymphocytes) but not on neutrophils (Valencia & Mills, 2006).

Several steps are involved in the recruitment of monocytes into vascular tissues: (i) initial selectin-dependent tethering and rolling, (ii) triggering of adhesion via chemokines and their receptors or through selectin binding to p-selectin glycoprotein ligand-1 (PSGL-1), (iii) integrin-dependent adhesion and adhesion strengthening by integrin clustering, and (iv) transmigration across endothelium (Galkina & Ley, 2007).

22

The interaction between surface integrins and endothelial adhesion molecules are leading to the migration of monocytes to the sites of inflammation via the process of firm adhesion and diapedesis (Daxecker et al., 2002). E-selectin and p-selectin are responsible for the contact between leucocytes and ECs during the inflammatory process (Lim et al., 1998). It has been reported that mice deficient in e-selectin and p-selectin receptors developed fewer fatty streak compared to controls and this indicates the importance of selectin interactions in atherogenesis (Dong et al., 1998).

It has been suggested that suitable therapeutics that can block leukocyte-endothelial interactions are the point of interest in the prevention of atherosclerosis (Lawson & Wolf 2009).

2.5   NUCLEAR FACTOR KAPPA β

The nuclear factor kappa B (NFκB) is the transcription factor which plays a role in immune and inflammatory responses through the regulation of genes encoding pro-inflammatory cytokines, adhesion molecules and chemokines (Kaileh & Sen, 2011). Under normal conditions, NFκB dimers are attached to inhibitory kappa B (IκB) proteins in the cytosolic compartment of the cell (Pamukcu et al., 2011).

NFκB pathway has been characterised into the canonical (classical) and non-canonical (alternative) pathways (Pamukcu et al., 2011). It has been reported that canonical pathway of NFκB activation is selectively involved in the upregulation of inflammation in atherosclerosis (Monaco et al., 2004). Inflammatory stimuli e.g. LPS activates the canonical pathway leading to the activation of the IκB kinase (IKK). Activation of IKK complex will then result in phosphorylation of IκB followed by the polyubiquitination and degradation by the proteosomes and release of NFκB (Chen, 2005). The free NFκB translocates to the nucleus and initiates transcription of target genes including pro-inflammatory and cell adhesion molecules (Chen, 2005).

NFκB1 p50 is one of the subunits of NFκB family that plays a crucial role in atherosclerosis (Kanters et al., 2004). Deletion of NFκB1 p50 receptors in mice has caused a significant reduction in lesion size and IL-6 (Kanters et al., 2004). It has been reported that p50 subunits are present in the nucleus of human atherosclerotic plaque cells (Monaco et al., 2004). NFκB p50 is generated by the proteolytic cleavage of precursor proteins p105 which are coded by the NFκB1 gene (Kanters et al., 2004). NFκB1 p50 binds to the kappa-B consensus sequence, located in the enhancer region of genes which involved in human response to acute phase reactions (Martinez et al., 2012). Targeting proteins that control the NF-κB signalling pathway that regulates the proteolysis of p105 may be useful for treatment of inflammatory diseases (Bienke & Lay, 2004).

2.6   SIGNAL TRANSDUCER AND ACTIVATOR OF TRANSCRIPTION-3

Other than the NFκB pathway, the signal transducers and activators of transcription (STATs) are also known to participate in the expression of adhesion molecule especially with regards to ICAM-1 (Yang et al., 2005). STATs are family of functionally related proteins that play a pivotal role in immune response (Chen et al., 2006). Among the STATs, signal transducer and activator of transcription protein 3 (STAT-3) can be activated by growth factors and cytokines i.e. IL-6 via the gp130 – Janus Kinase (JAK) pathway (Coccia et al., 1999). STAT-3 has been described as a factor in acute phase reaction after induction by IL-6 (Yang et al., 2005).

In response to IL-6, JAK 2 (gp130) is activated and followed by the phoshorylation of STAT-3 monomers (Tyr705 and Ser727). Phosphorylation of STAT-3 allows dimerization and translocation into to the nucleus, where it binds to IL-6 response elements (IRE) and regulates gene expression (Roy et al., 2001; Schuringa et al., 2001). In the ischaemic reperfusion, it has been reported that the specificity protein 1 (sp1) - STAT3 complex play an important role in the upregulation of ICAM-1. ECs treated with IL-6 increased the expression of ICAM-1 through STAT-3 signaling pathway (Chen et al., 2006).

2.7 ENDOTHELIAL NITRIC OXIDE SYNTHASE

Endothelial nitric oxide synthase (eNOS) is expressed in vascular ECs, especially at the endothelial layer of medium to large sized blood vessel (Fish et al., 2005). eNOS play an important role in the nitric oxide (NO) production by ECs (Hickey, 2001). Endothelium derived NO function as a potent vasodilator in the vasculature where the balance between NO and endothelium-derived vasoconstrictors and the sympathetic nervous system maintains blood vessel tone and pressure (Vallence & Chan, 2001). NO modulates vascular tone, inhibits platelet function, prevents adhesion of leukocytes and reduces proliferation of the intima (Forstermann, 2010). NO also functions as an anti-inflammatory agent and depresses leukocyte adhesion (Kuhlencordt et al., 2004). NO modulates leukocyte-endothelial cell activation through direct effect of NO on the regulation of cytokines and adhesion molecule expression by the transcription factor NFκB (Spiecker et al., 1997). NO induces transcription of IκBα, an inhibitor of NFκB thus stabilizing the inhibitory NFκB/ IκBα complex in the cytosol (Peng et al., 1995). Another protective effect of NO is that it can protect cells from oxidative stress because NO interacts rapidly with superoxide, a pro-adhesive molecule (Kuhlencordt et al., 2004).

eNOS generally has protective effects within the cardiovascular system (Fish et al., 2005). It has been indicated that eNOS plays a protective role in cerebral ischemia by preserving cerebral blood flow in eNOS knockout mice (Huang & Lo, 1998). Dramatic decrease of eNOS can occur during early stages of atherosclerosis leading to NO reduction (Zhang et al., 2010).

eNOS mediated NO production upon the conversion of L-arginine to L-citrulline and eNOS activity is modulated by agonists of diverse G-protein-coupled cell surface receptors and by physical stimuli such as haemodynamic shear stress (Shaul, 2003). It has been reported that TNF-α is a powerful modulator of eNOS mRNA expression (Nishida et al., 1992). IL-6 can lead to decrease of eNOS expression and contributes to the attenuation of NO production and progression of atherosclerosis (Saura et al., 2006).

It has been found that localized inflammatory reactions and enhanced local oxidative stress lead to abnormal endothelium-dependent relaxation at both coronary conduit and resistance arteries, myocardial hypertrophy and coronary artery restenosis (Pendyala et al., 2009). Altered NO production and/or bioavailability have been linked to several diverse disorders such as hypertension, hypercholesterolemia, diabetes, and heart failure (Harrison, 1997).

2.8   ATHEROSCLEROSIS

Atherosclerosis is the main underlying cause of CAD and other cardiovascular diseases including myocardium infarction (MI), stable angina and unstable angina (Lewis et al., 2011). It is a slowly progressing disease arising from the combination of chronic inflammation and endothelial activation leading to the formation of fatty and fibrous lessions in the walls of large and medium-sized arteries (Hansson & Hermansson, 2011). The progression of atherosclerosis is illustrated in Figure 2.4. Various epidemiological studies have shown a significant link between coronary artery disease (CAD) and chronic inflammatory diseases (Klingenberg & Hansson, 2009). Complications due to atherosclerosis account for the majority of adult illnesses and deaths worldwide each year with approximately 16.7 million people around the world (Gersh et al., 2010). Furthermore, cardiovascular disease is projected to be the number one killer globally by 2020 (Klingenberg & Hansson, 2009). The first clinical manifestation of cardiovascular disease often arises in the stage of well-developed atherosclerosis (Poredos, 2011).

Various risk factors have been identified in the pathogenesis of atherosclerosis including hypertension, smoking, increased concentrations of low density lipoprotein plasma Cholesterol (LDL-c), diabetes, obesity, age and gender (male) (Lusis, 2000). Other than that, stimulants (LPS and ox-LDL) and environment stressors (microgravity, hypergravity and mechanical stress) may also cause endothelial injury and trigger an inflammatory response (Lewis et al., 2011). Subsequently endothelial activation may occur, leading to increase in vascular permeability, adhesion of monocytes and expression of pro-coagulant molecules (Lawson & Wolf, 2009). Continuous inflammation and endothelial activation can facilitate the infiltration of atherogenic lipoproteins and the entry of monocytes and lymphocytes into the sub-endothelial space (Lawson & Wolf, 2009). The activation of these macrophages and lymphocytes lead to the release of hydrolytic enzymes, cytokines, chemokines and

26

growth factors. This will activate the classical and alternative complement pathway of the immune system,

FIGURE 2.4

**Progression of Atherosclerosis in the Blood Vessels. CAD - Coronary Artery Disease
Source: Klingenberg & Hansson (2009)**

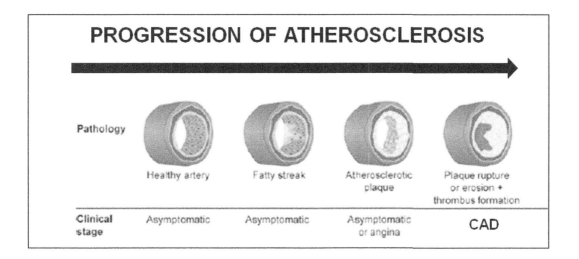

increase cell permeability and platelet activation, stimulate the proliferation and migration of smooth muscle cells and promote fatty-fibrous tissue deposition into the vessel wall leading to the formation and progression of fatty - fibrous plaques (Lusis, 2000).

The lesions may evolve to contain large amounts of lipids and if it becomes unstable or rupture, it may result in thrombotic occlusion of the overlying endothelium, leading to clinical events such as acute MI, stroke and acute coronary syndrome (Koenig & Khuseyinova, 2007). The pathogenesis of atherosclerosis is presented in diagram in Figure 2.5.

Biomarkers for early detection of atherosclerosis are important, so that life style changes or intervention can be effective before atherosclerosis progresses and lead to MI or stroke. Therefore, detection of biomarkers of atherosclerosis is important for the prevention of progression of atherosclerosis and cardiovascular events in view that the development of atherosclerosis plaques is asymptomatic and usually takes many decades (Poredos, 2011). IL-6, TNF-α, ICAM-1, VCAM-1 and e-selectin have been suggested as potential early biomarkers of atherosclerosis (Fan & Watanabe, 2003). This suggestion is based on several prospective epidemiological studies that have found increased vascular risk in association with increased basal levels of the above biomarkers (Ridker et al., 2000). Furthermore, elevated levels of inflammatory mediators and adhesion molecules have been indicated in subjects with atherosclerosis (Poredos, 2011).

FIGURE 2.5

Pathogenesis of Atherosclerosis

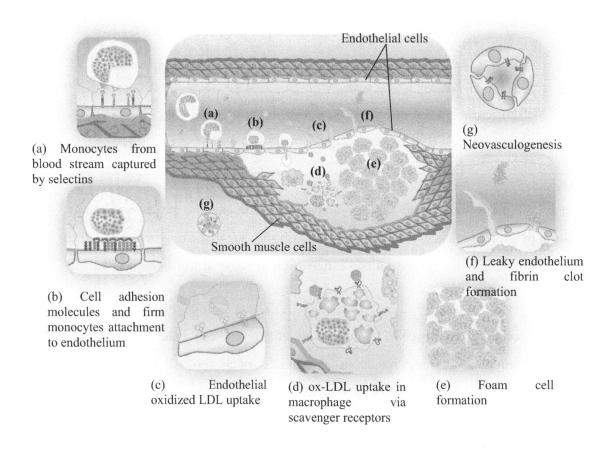

(a) Monocytes from blood stream captured by selectins

(b) Cell adhesion molecules and firm monocytes attachment to endothelium

(c) Endothelial oxidized LDL uptake

(d) ox-LDL uptake in macrophage via scavenger receptors

(e) Foam cell formation

(f) Leaky endothelium and fibrin clot formation

(g) Neovasculogenesis

Elevated LDL and stimulants (e.g. lipopolysaccharides) stimulate ECs to trigger the inflammatory response. Selectins (e.g. e-selectin) and adhesion molecules facilitate the recruitment of monocytes from circulation through the endothelial membrane and increase the permeability of endothelium capturing more LDL into the sub-endothelial space. Monocytes differentiated into macrophages and uptake ox-LDL via scavenger receptor. Unregulated uptake of ox-LDL by macrophages leads to formation of lipid-filled foam cells. Foam cells expressed inflammatory cytokines continuing cycle of inflammation and lipoprotein modification. Following the accumulation of lipid laden macrophage, smooth muscle cells migrate into the lipid layer. Significant build-up leads to a necrotic lipid core surrounded by fibrous cap. Compromised endothelial expose

basement membrane to thrombosis, forming fibrin clots. Neovasculogenesis take place to fulfil the increased metabolic demand of the cells in the growing plaque in the media extend into the media. The plaque may become unstable or rupture resulting in thrombotic occlusion of the overlying endothelium, leading to clinical events such as heart attack, stroke and acute coronary syndrome.
Source: Lewis et al., (2011).

CHAPTER THREE
METHODOLOGY

3.1   MATERIALS

Tocotrienol enriched mixed fraction (TEMF) was provided by Golden Hope Jomalina Sdn. Bhd. Malaysia (Table 3.1). Pure isomers of α-, β-, γ- and δ-TCT and α-TOC (> 97 %) were provided by Davos Lifesciences, Singapore. Medium 200 and low serum growth supplements (LSGS) were obtained from Cascade Biologics, USA. RPMI-1640 medium (with glutamax-I and HEPES), L-glutamine and fetal bovine serum (FBS) were purchased from Gibco-Life Technologies, USA. Penicillin/streptomycin was purchased from PAA laboratories, Austria. [3-(4, 5-Dimethylthiazol-2-yl)]-2, 5-diphenyltetrazolium bromide (MTT) and dimethyl sulfoxide (DMSO) was purchased from Fluka, Germany. Accutase was purchased from ICN Biomedical, USA. Phosphate buffer saline (PBS) was obtained from MP Biomedicals, France. Rose Bengal was obtained from Sigma Aldrich, USA. ELISA test kits for IL6, TNF-α, sICAM-1, sVCAM-1 and E-selectin were purchased from Bender Medsystems, Austria. NFκB binding assay kit was obtained from Cayman Chemicals, USA. Quantikine eNOS immunoassay kit was manufactured by R&D BioSystems (USA). RNA extraction kit and Sensiscript Reverse Transcription kit was manufactured by Qiagen, USA. Agilent RNA 6000 Pico was manufactured by Agilent Technologies, Germany. Primers for Quantitative real time (qPCR) assay were produced by First BASE Laboratories, Malaysia. SYBR Green for qPCR assay was obtained from Bio-Rad Laboratories, Hercules, California. All chemicals used in this assay were tissue culture grade.

3.2   CELL CULTURE

Human umbilical vein endothelial cells (HUVECs) were purchased from Cascade Biologics, USA. HUVECs were cultured in medium 200 supplemented with LSGS in a humidified incubator set at 37 °C and 5 % carbon dioxide (CO_2) until confluent. Cells were grown in 25 cm^2 culture flasks (BD Falcon, UK). Cells were harvested by cell detachment solution (Accutase) and sub-cultivation ratio was 1:3 (culture: medium). All chemicals used in this assay were tissue culture grade.

TABLE 3.1

The Composition of Tocotrienol-Enriched Mixed Fraction (TEMF)

Vitamin E components	Percentage, %	Weight (mg/g)
α- tocopherol	34.5	233.4
α - tocotrienol	26.7	180.7
β - tocotrienol	2.2	14.6
γ - tocotrienol	22.8	154.5
δ - tocotrienol	13.8	93.3
Total	100	676.5

3.3 PREPARATION OF DIFFERENT CONCENTRATIONS OF TEMF AND PURE TCT ISOMERS IN CELL CULTURE MEDIUM

A stock solution of TEMF or pure α, β, γ, δ-TCT isomers or α-TOC were firstly prepared in absolute ethanol and stored at -80 °C for not more than three days. The sample stocks were then mixed with FBS at a ratio of 1:20 and incubated at 37°C for 15 minutes during which time a brief vortex was conducted every five minutes. After that, the working solution of each samples were prepared in RPMI-1640 culture medium. These working solution were further diluted with RPMI-1640 to obtain the desired concentrations needed in each assay. The final ethanol concentration in each TEMF or pure α, β, γ, δ-TCT isomers or α-TOC and controls (unstimulated and LPS alone) in the assay plate were 0.004 %. The final FBS concentrations in all samples were standardized to 8 %.

3.4 CELL CYTOTOXICITY ASSAY

At the beginning, TEMF was first tested for its toxicity concentrations against HUVECs by using [3-(4, 5-Dimethylthiazol-2-yl)]-2, 5-diphenyltetrazolium bromide] metabolic (MTT) assay (Mosmann, 1983). MTT is cleaved to formazan by the succinate-tetrazolium reductase system, which belongs to the mitochondrial respiratory chain and is active in living cells. Mitochondrial electron transport plays a major role in the cellular reduction of MTT and occurs mostly in the cytoplasm. Briefly, 100 μl of 1×10^5 cells/ml were seeded into 96-well micro titer plates in the presence of varying concentrations of TEMF (0.3 – 100 μM, 0.2 - 54.1 μg/ml) prior to incubation for 24 hours in a humidified incubator set at 37 °C and 5 % CO_2. Control wells of untreated cell populations were also included. A volume of 20 μl of MTT solution [5 mg MTT in 1 ml phosphate buffer saline (PBS)] was added to each well, followed by 4 hours incubation at 37 °C. Then, 170 μl of the medium was removed from each well before the addition of 100 μl of DMSO to solubilize the formazan crystal formed after incubation with MTT. The plate was then incubated at room temperature for 30-50 minutes. The absorbance of each well was measured at 550 nm wavelength using a microplate reader (Micro Quant, Biotek Instruments Inc, USA).

3.5 SOLUBLE PROTEIN EXPRESSION OF INFLAMMATION AND ENDOTHELIAL ACTIVATION BIOMARKERS IN ENDOTHELIAL CELLS

The confluent HUVECs grown in 75 cm^2 culture flasks were washed with PBS and harvested by cell detachment solution (Accutase). After that, the cells were cultured into six-well culture plates until confluence. The cells were then washed twice with prewarmed PBS and a volume of 1000 μl of RPMI-1640 medium containing 25 mmol/l HEPES, 2 mmol/l glutamax-I, 10 % FBS and antibiotics were added. Cells were stimulated with LPS (1 μg/ml) and different concentrations of TEMF (0.3 - 10 μM) were added prior to the incubation in a CO_2 incubator for 16 hours. At the end of the incubation period, a volume of 900 μl of the supernatant in each well was centrifuged at 1200 rpm for five minutes). Thereafter, three portions of 190 μl from each sample were stored at -80 °C until used. Concentrations of soluble inflammation markers in supernatant of HUVECs were determined using the ELISA standard kit (Bender Med System, Vienna, Austria). Tests were performed according to the instructions provided by the manufacturer. Surface levels of inflammation markers in each cell culture supernatant were performed in triplicates. Briefly, an amount of 100 μl aliquots of cell culture media was transferred to anti e-selectin, p-selectin, sICAM-1, sVCAM-1 or IL-6 antibody-coated wells. The peroxidase-conjugated secondary polyclonal antibody was added into each well. After three times washing steps, substrate solution was then added into each well and reaction was allowed to develop for 30 minutes. The colour development was stopped and absorbance was measured at 405 nm using a microplate reader (Tecan Safire, Männedorf, Switzerland).

3.6   MONOCYTES BINDING ASSAY

Firstly, HUVECs were seeded in 96-well micro titer plates at a seeding density of 1 X 10^5 cells/ml and incubated overnight in a humidified incubator set at 37 °C and 5 % CO_2. HUVECs were then treated with varying concentrations of TEMF or α, β, γ, δ-TCT isomers or α-TOC (0.3 – 100 µM) together with LPS (1 µg/ml) prior to incubation for 16 hours in a humidified incubator set at 37 °C and 5 % CO_2. After that, an amount of 0.5 X 10^6 ml human monocytic cells (U937) was added into each well and kept for an hour in a humidified incubator set at 37 °C and 5 % CO_2. At the end of incubation, the unbound U937 was washed away with RPMI-1640. Then, 100 µl of 0.25 % Rose Bengal in PBS was added into each well and incubated for 10 minutes in room temperature. Excess stain were washed away for three times with PBS containing 10 % FBS. After washing,   200 µl of ethanol: PBS (1:1 v/v) solution was added into each well and incubated for an hour at room temperature. After incubation, the absorbance in each well was read at 570 nm wavelength with a microplate reader (Tecan Safire, Männedorf, Switzerland)

3.7   NFκB BINDING ASSAY

HUVECs in 25 cm^2 culture flasks were treated with different concentrations of TEMF or α, β, γ, δ-TCT isomers or α-TOC together with LPS (1 µg/ml) for 16 hours in CO_2 incubator set at 37 °C. After incubation, HUVECs were harvested with cell detachment solution (Accutase) and transferred into pre-chilled 15 ml centrifuge tubes to perform nuclear extraction process. At the beginning, the cells suspension was centrifuged at 300 g for five minutes. The cell pellets were resuspended in five ml ice cold PBS/Phosphate inhibitor solution and centrifuged at 300g for five minutes at 4 °C. An amount of 500 µl of ice cold 1x hypotonic buffer was added into the cell pellets and transferred into a pre-chilled 1.5 microcentrifuge tube. The cells were allowed to swell by incubating it on ice for 15 minutes. After that, 100 μl of 10 % Nonidet P-40 assay reagent was added and centrifuged for 30 seconds at 4 °C in a microcentrifuge. The cell pallets were resuspended in 50 μl ice-cold complete nuclear extraction buffer containing protease and phosphatase inhibitors. The tubes were vortexed for 15 seconds at the highest setting and incubated on a shaking platform for 15 minutes. The tubes were then vortexed for another 30 seconds and incubated on a shaking platform for 15 an additional of 15 minutes. Cells were centrifuged at 14,000 g for ten minutes at 4 °C. The supernatant containing nuclear extract was collected and aliquot into several clean microtubes. The samples were flash frozen and kept in -80 °C until analysis. Quantification of NFκB (p50) protein binding in nuclear extract was performed by ELISA method according to the manufacturer instruction manual (Cayman Chemicals). The nuclear extracts at 500 μg concentration for every sample were added into each well coated with consensus double stranded DNA (dsDNA) sequence. Transcription factor in the nuclear extracts were allowed to bind with the dsDNA overnight at 4 °C. After incubation, the plate was washed to remove unbound reagents. Then primary antibody that binds to transcriptional factor was added into each well. After washing, the secondary antibody goat anti-rabbit horseradish peroxidase (HRP) conjugate was added to bind with primary antibody. After washing, the developing solution was added into each well and incubated on a platform shaker for 45 minutes. At the end of incubation, stop solution was added into each well. The absorbance in each well was measured at 450 nm with a microplate reader (Tecan Safire, Männedorf, Switzerland).

3.8   QUANTIFICATION OF eNOS PROTEIN LEVEL IN CELL LYSATES

HUVECs in 25 cm^2 culture flask were treated with   different concentrations of TEMF or α, β, γ, δ-TCT isomers or α-TOC   (0.3 – 10 μM) together with LPS (1 μg/ml) for 16 hours in CO_2 incubator set at 37 °C. After incubation, HUVECs were harvested with cell detachment solution (Accutase) and transferred into pre-chilled 15 ml centrifuge tube. The cells suspension was centrifuge at 1100 rpm for five minutes. The supernatant were discarded gently. After that, the cell pallet was washed twice with saline solution by centrifugation at 1100 rpm for five minutes. The supernatant were then discarded gently. The cells lysis buffer (4 °C) was added into the cell pellet and centrifuged at 1100 rpm for five minutes. The supernatant was collected and preceded with eNOS immunoassay. All reagents and samples for this assay were thawed at room temperature prior to use. Firstly, seven different concentration of eNOS standard ranging from 4000 to 62.5 pg/ml were prepared according to instruction manual. In the ELISA plat, 100 µl of assay diluents was added into each well. Then 100 µl of standard, samples and controls were added into their assigned wells. The plate was sealed and incubated for two hours at room temperature on platform shaker set at 500 rpm. After washing, 200 µl of eNOS conjugate was added into each well and incubate for another two hours in room temperature on platform shaker set at 500 rpm. After washing, 200 µl of substrate solution was added into each well and incubated for 30 minutes at room temperature on the bench top. At the end of incubation, 50 µl of stop solution was added into each well. The optical density of each well was determined using a microplate reader (Tecan Safire, Männedorf, Switzerland) set at 450 nm and reference wavelength at 570 nm.

3.9 IL-6, TNF-α, ICAM-1, VCAM-1, E-SELECTIN, NFκB AND eNOS GENE EXPRESSION BY QUANTITATIVE REAL TIME PCR

HUVECs in 25 cm^2 culture flask were treated with different concentrations of TEMF or α, β, γ, δ-TCT isomers or α-TOC (0.3 – 10 µM) together with LPS (1 µg/ml) for 16 hours in CO_2 incubator set at 37 °C. After incubation, HUVECs were harvested with cell detachment solution (Accutase). The cell pellets were obtained by centrifugation at 1100 rpm for 5 minutes. The gene expression analysis was carried out by qPCR assay according to the similar method described in Chapter 3.

3.10 STATISTICAL ANALYSIS

Results are expressed as mean $\pm$ SD. Analysis of variance (ANOVA) was performed to assess overall differences between the different treatments. Independent T-test was performed to compare the differences between the two groups of treatment. All data was analysed by a statistical package programme, SPSS version 16.0. Level of significance was set at $p < 0.05$.

CHAPTER FOUR
RESULTS

4.1 EFFECTS OF TEMF ON CELL VIABILITY

Effects of varying concentrations of tocotrienol on cell viability were observed by MTT assay. TEMF greater than 10 μM showed reduced cell viability as when compared to control untreated cell population (Figure 4.1). As a result, TEMF no greater than 10 μM were used to treat the cells for the experiments.

4.2 EFFECTS OF TEMF ON SOLUBLE PROTEIN EXPRESSION OF CYTOKINE (IL-6 AND TNF-α AND ADHESION MOLECULES (ICAM-1, VCAM-1 AND E-SELECTIN) IN LPS-STIMULATED HUVECs

There was an increment of IL-6 soluble protein concentration in HUVECs treated with LPS compared to the unstimulated cells (1900.0 $\pm$ 56.9 vs. 171.5 $\pm$ 1.0 pg/ml, $p<0.0001$. The addition of TEMF in LPS stimulated cells reduced the production of IL-6 throughout all concentrations [Figure 4.2 (a)]. However, the reduction of IL-6 by TEMF was only significant at 0.3 μM (the lowest concentration) compared to HUVECs incubated with LPS alone (933.3 $\pm$ 188.6 vs. 1900.0 $\pm$ 56.9 pg/ml, $p< 0.05$). Figure 4.2 (b) shows the percentage inhibition of TEMF throughout all concentrations with the highest inhibition of 56.0 $\pm$ 12.0 % TEMF at the 0.3 μM which is at the lowest concentration

LPS treatment in HUVECs cells lead to induction of TNF-α compared to the level of unstimulated HUVECs (62.3 $\pm$ 0.6 vs. 31.9 $\pm$ 2.7 pg/ml, $p<0.01$). The addition of TEMF in LPS stimulated HUVECs did not significantly reduce the production of TNF-α throughout all concentrations [Figure 4.3 (a)]. TEMF at 1.3 μM had the greatest TNF-α concentration but it was not statistically significant when compared to LPS alone (54.2 $\pm$ 0.0 vs. 62.3 $\pm$ 0.6 pg/ml, NS). Figure 4.3 (b) shows the percentage inhibition of TNF-α by TEMF (0.3 μM – 10 μM) in LPS stimulated HUVECs. The highest TNF-α percentage of inhibition was shown by TEMF at 1.3 μM (12.9 $\pm$ 0.0 %).

FIGURE 4.1

Effects of TEMF on Cell Viability. HUVECs Were Grown in 96 Well Microplate Until Confluent. Cells Were Pretreated With Various Concentrations of TEMF (0.3 – 100 μM) for 24 hours. After Pretreatment, Cells Were Subjected to the MTT Cytotoxicity Assay. Data are Expressed as Percentage of Cell Viability. Data are Expressed as Mean ± SD (n=3)

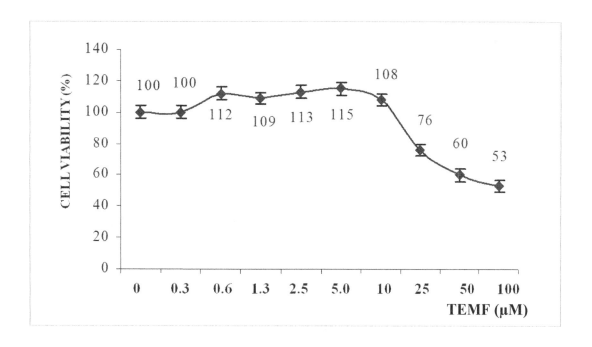

FIGURE 4.2 (a)

Effects of TEMF (0.3 - 10 μM) on the IL-6 Soluble Protein Expression in LPS Stimulated HUVECs. Prior to Incubation, IL-6 Protein Expression in the Supernatant Was Measured by ELISA. Results are Expressed as IL-6 Concentration (pg/ml). Data are Expressed as Mean ± SD (n=3). * p<0.05 and **** p< 0.0001 Compared to HUVECs Incubated with LPS Alone

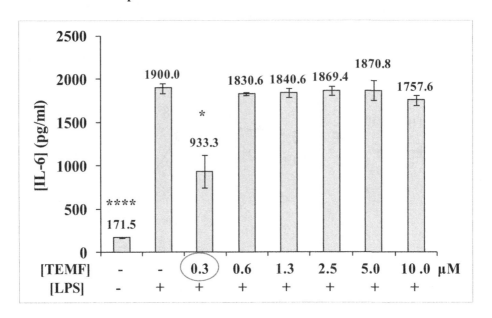

FIGURE 4.2 (b)

% Inhibition of Soluble IL-6 Protein Expression By Various Concentrations of TEMF (0.3 - 10 μM) over LPS Stimulated HUVECs. Varying Concentrations of TEMF Were Added to the HUVECs Together With LPS (1 μg/ml) and Incubated in a Humidified Incubator Set at 37 °C and 5 % CO_2 for 16 hours. Data are Expressed as Mean ± SD (n=3). ANOVA p<0.0001.

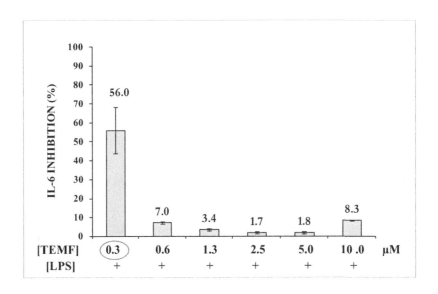

FIGURE 4.3 (a):

Effects of TEMF (0.3 – 10 μM) on the TNF-α Soluble Protein Expression in LPS Stimulated HUVECs. Prior to Incubation, TNF-α Protein Expression in the Supernatant was Measured by ELISA. Results are Expressed as TNF-α Concentration (pg/ml). Data are Expressed as Mean ± SD (n=3). ** p<0.01 Compared to HUVECs Incubated with LPS Alone.

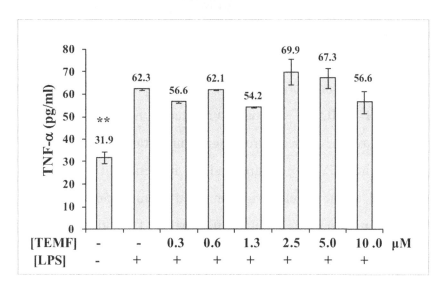

FIGURE 4.3 (b)

% Inhibition of Soluble TNF-α Protein Concentration by Various Concentrations of TEMF (0.3 - 10 μM) over LPS Stimulated HUVECs. Varying Concentrations of TEMF were Added to the HUVECs Together with LPS (1 μg/ml) and Incubated in a Humidified Incubator set at 37 °C and 5 % CO$_2$ for 16 hours. Data are Expressed as Mean ± SD (n=3). ANOVA, NS.

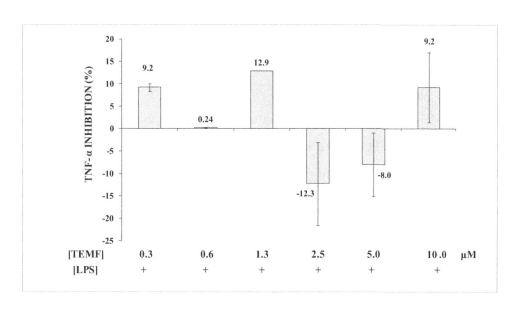

LPS treatment in HUVECs had significantly increased the production of soluble ICAM-1 (sICAM-1) compared to those unstimulated HUVECs (10643.5 ± 19.7 vs. 2022.3 ± 39.4 pg/ml, $p<0.0001$). Presence of varying concentrations of TEMF ($0.3 - 10$ µM) in HUVECs stimulated with LPS inhibits production of sICAM-1 ($p<0.0001$) as illustrated in Figure 4.4 (a). TEMF at the concentration of 1.3 µM showed the lowest production of sICAM in LPS stimulated cultures (5908.1 ± 256.1 vs. 10643.5 ± 19.7 pg/ml, $p<0.01$). Figure 4.4 (b) shows the significant inhibition of sICAM-1 across all concentrations and the percentage inhibition of varying concentrations of TEMF in HUVECs culture stimulated with LPS, at which TEMF at 1.3 µM concentration gave the highest percentage of inhibition (54.9 ± 2.6 %).

LPS treatment in HUVECs culture leads to induction of soluble VCAM-1 (sVCAM-1) compared to the level of unstimulated culture (5689.7 ± 278.7 vs. 3559.0 ± 156.7 pg/ml, $p<0.01$). The addition of TEMF in LPS stimulated HUVECs culture reduced the production of sVCAM-1 throughout all concentrations, $p<0.0001$ [Figure 4.5 (a)]. TEMF at 5 µM gave the greatest reduction of sVCAM-1 compared cultures incubated with LPS alone (4088.7 ± 104.5 vs. 5689.7 ± 278.7 pg/ml ($p< 0.01$). Figure 4.5 (b) shows significant inhibition of sVCAM-1 across all concentrations with the highest inhibition showed by TEMF at 5 µM concentration (75.0 ± 3.8 %).

LPS at the concentration of 1 µg/ml significantly increased the production of e-selectin compared to unstimulated HUVECs (7358.4 ± 303.2 vs. 2381.3 ± 129.9 pg/ml, $p<0.0001$). TEMF has been shown to inhibit production of selectin in LPS stimulated HUVECs culture throughout all concentrations ($p<0.0001$) [Figure 4.6 (a)]. The lowest production of e-selectin has been shown in culture incubated with 1.3 µM of TEMF together with LPS when compared to culture incubated with LPS alone (2955.6 ± 164.4 vs. 7358.4 ± 303.2 pg/ml, $p<0.01$). Percentage inhibitions of varying concentrations of TEMF are shown in Figure 4.6 (b). TEMF at the 0.3 µM concentrations was shown to have highest percentage inhibition of e-selectin (88.4 ± 1.7 %).

FIGURE 4.4 (a)

Effects of TEMF (0.3 - 10 μM) on the sICAM-1 Protein Expression in LPS Stimulated HUVECs. Prior to Incubation, sICAM-1 Protein Expression in the supernatant was measured by ELISA. Results are Expressed as sICAM-1 Concentration (pg/ml). Data are Expressed as Mean $\pm$ SD (n=3). * p<0.05, ** p<0.01 and **** p<0.0001 Compared to HUVECs Incubated with LPS alone.

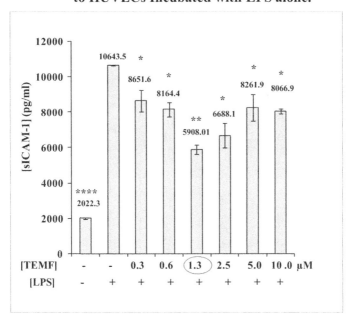

FIGURE 4.4 (b)

% Inhibition of Soluble ICAM-1 Protein Concentration by Various Concentrations of TEMF (0.3 - 10 μM) over LPS Stimulated HUVECs. Varying Concentrations of TEMF Were Added to the HUVECs Together with LPS (1 μg/ml) and Incubated in a Humidified Incubator set at 37 °C and 5 % CO_2 for 16 hours. Data are Expressed as Mean $\pm$ SD (n=3). ANOVA, p<0.0001.

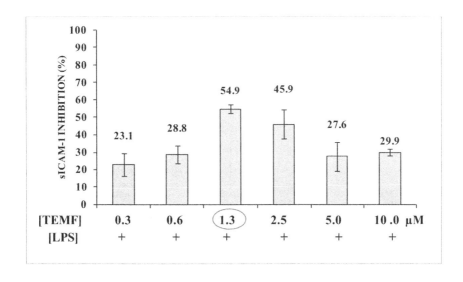

FIGURE 4.5 (a)

Effects of TEMF (0.3 - 10 μM) on the sVCAM-1 Protein Expression in LPS Stimulated HUVECs. Prior to Incubation, sVCAM-1 Protein Expression in the Supernatant Was Measured by ELISA. Results are Expressed as sVCAM-1 Concentration (pg/ml). Data Are Expressed as Mean ± SD (n=3). * p<0.05, ** p<0.01 and *** p<0.001 Compared to HUVECs incubated with LPS Alone

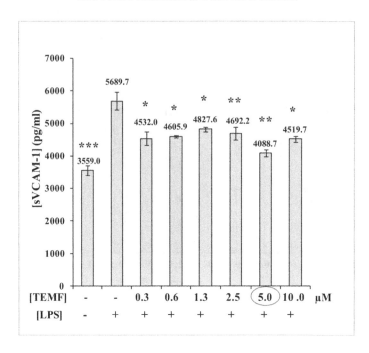

FIGURE 4.5 (b)

% Inhibition of Soluble VCAM-1 Protein Concentration by Various Concentrations of TEMF (0.3 - 10 μM) over LPS Stimulated HUVECs. Varying Concentrations of TEMF Were Added to the HUVECs Together With LPS (1 μg/ml) and Incubated in a Humidified Incubator Set at 37 °C and 5 % CO₂ for 16 Hours. Data are Expressed as Mean ± SD (n=3). ANOVA, p<0.0001

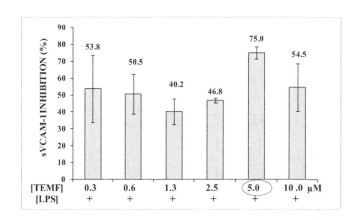

FIGURE 4.6 (a)

Effects of TEMF (0.3 - 10 μM) on the E-selectin Protein Expression in LPS stimulated HUVECs. Prior to Incubation, e-selectin Protein Expression in the Supernatant Was Measured by ELISA. Results are Expressed as E-selectin Concentration (pg/ml). Data are Expressed as Mean ± SD (n=3). * p<0.05, ** p<0.01 and *** p<0.001 Compared to HUVECs Incubated With LPS Alone

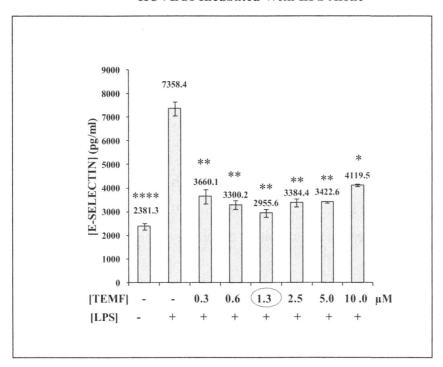

FIGURE 4.6 (b)

% Inhibition of Soluble E-selectin Protein Concentration by Various Concentrations of TEMF (0.3 - 10 μM) over LPS Stimulated HUVECS. Varying Concentrations of TEMF Were Added to the HUVECs Together with LPS (1 μg/ml) and Incubated in a Humidified Incubator Set at 37 °C and 5 % CO$_2$ for 16 Hours. Data Are Expressed as Mean ± SD (n=3). ANOVA, p<0.0001

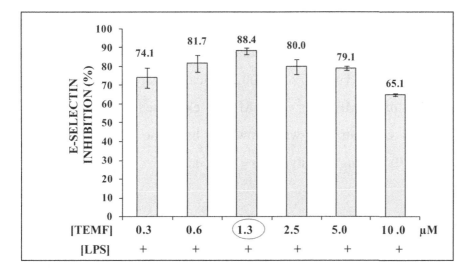

4.3 EFFECTS OF TEMF ON MONOCYTES BINDING ACTIVITY IN LPS-STIMULATED HUVECS

Monocytes binding activity with the endothelial cells were measured by Rose Bengal Staining. Increment of monocytes binding to the endothelial cells is a key event to the pathogenesis of atherosclerosis. Therefore the effects of TEMF on the ability of monocytes to bind to HUVEC cells were investigated. LPS treatment of HUVECs significantly increased monocyte binding activity compared to unstimulated HUVECs ($p < 0.05$). The addition of TEMF (0.3- 10 μM) to LPS stimulated HUVECs culture reduced monocyte binding activity, $p < 0.05$ [Figure 4.7 (a)]. TEMF at 0.3 μM showed the lowest monocytes binding activity compared to LPS alone (0.80 $\pm$ 0.01 vs. 2.6 $\pm$ 0.01 fold change, $p < 0.05$). Percentage inhibitions of varying concentrations of TEMF are expressed in Figure 4.7 (b). TEMF at the 0.3 μM concentrations was shown to have the highest percentage inhibition of monocyte binding activity (69.6 $\pm$ 0.8 %).

4.4 EFFECTS OF TEMF ON NFκB (p50) TRANSCRIPTION FACTOR DNA BINDING ACTIVITY IN LPS-STIMULATED HUVECS

LPS treatment in HUVECs significantly increased the NFκB (p50) transcription factor DNA binding activity ($p < 0.001$). Figure 4.8 (a) shows the effects of TEMF (0.3-10 μM) on the NFκB transcription factor DNA binding activity in LPS stimulated HUVECs. TEMF throughout all concentrations (0.3 - 10 μM) lead to reduction of NFκB (p50) binding activity in LPS stimulated HUVECs ($p < 0.0001$). NFκB (p50) binding activity was optimally reduced by TEMF at 0.6 μM compared to LPS alone [0.118 $\pm$ 0.004 vs. 0.172 $\pm$ 0.002 optical density (OD), $p < 0.0001$). Percentage inhibitions of TEMF (0.3 - 10 μM) are expressed in Figure 4.8 (b). TEMF at the 0.6 μM concentration was shown to have the highest percentage inhibition of NFκB (p50) binding activity (69.6 $\pm$ 0.8 %).

FIGURE 4.7 (a)

Effects of TEMF (0.3 - 10 μM) on the Monocytes Binding Activity in LPS Stimulated HUVECs. Prior to Incubation, Cells were Subjected to the Monocytes Binding Assay. Data are Expressed as Mean $\pm$ SD (n=3). * p<0.05, ** p<0.01 and *** p<0.001 Compared to HUVECs Incubated with LPS alone

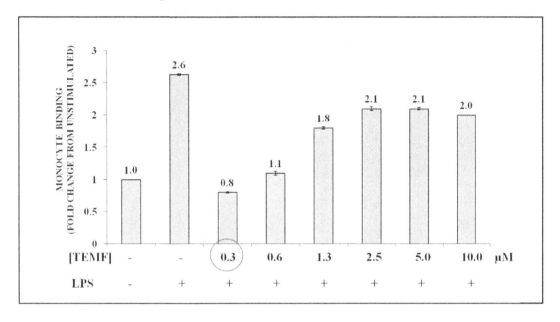

FIGURE 4.7 (b)

% Inhibition of Monocytes Binding Activity by Various Concentrations of TEMF (0.3 - 10 μM) over LPS stimulated HUVECs. Varying Concentrations of TEMF Were Added to the HUVECs Together with LPS (1 μg/ml) and Incubated in a Humidified Incubator Set at 37 °C and 5 % CO_2 for 16 Hours. Data are Expressed as Mean $\pm$ SD (n=3). ANOVA p<0.0001

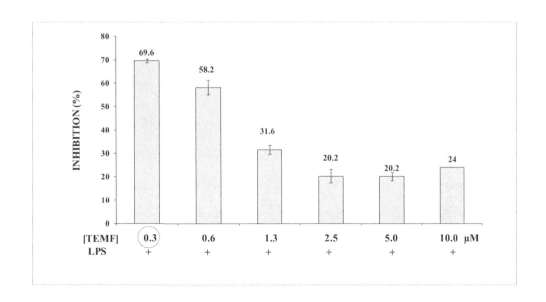

FIGURE 4.8 (a):

Effects of TEMF (0.3 - 10μM) on the NFκB Binding Activity in LPS Stimulated HUVECs. Prior to Incubation, Nuclear Extracts Were Isolated and Level of NFκB Binding Activity Was Measured by NFκB p50 Transcription Factor Assay kit. Data are expressed as mean ± SD (n=3). * p<0.05, ** p<0.01 and **** p< 0.0001 Compared to HUVECs Incubated with LPS alone

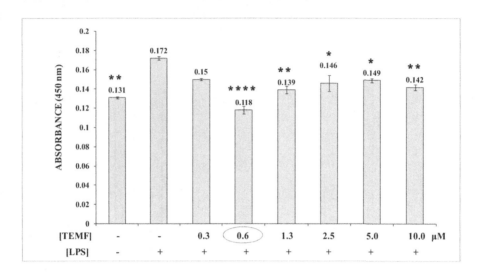

FIGURE 4.8 (b):

% Inhibition of NFκB Activity by Various Concentrations of TEMF (0.3 - 10 μM) over LPS Stimulated HUVECs. Varying Concentrations of TEMF were Added to the HUVECs Together with LPS (1 μg/ml) and Incubated in a Humidified Incubator Set at 37 °C and 5 % CO_2 for 16 Hours. Data are Expressed as Mean ± SD (n=3). ANOVA p<0.0001

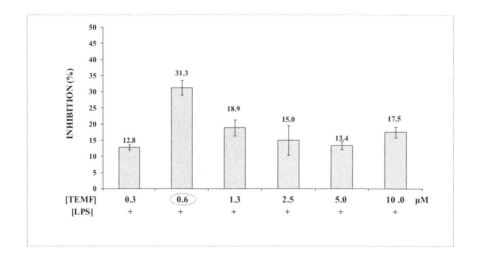

4.5 EFFECTS OF TEMF ON eNOS PROTEIN EXPRESSION IN LPS-STIMULATED HUVECs

Endothelial nitric oxide synthase (eNOS) expression is significantly decreased by LPS treatment compared to unstimulated HUVECs ($p < 0.05$). Figure 4.9 (a) shows the effects of TEMF (0.3 - 10 μM) on the eNOS protein expression in LPS stimulated HUVECs. TEMF at 0.6 μM showed the highest eNOS protein expression compared to LPS alone (3439.3 $\pm$ 19.8 vs. 2978.8 $\pm$ 6.7 pg/ml, $p < 0.0001$). Figure 4.9 (b) illustrates the percentage increment of eNOS protein expression by TEMF (0.3 - 10 μM) over LPS stimulated HUVECs. The highest percentage increment of eNOS was expressed by TEMF at 0.6 μM with 17.3 % of increment over LPS stimulated HUVECs.

4.6 EFFECTS OF TEMF ON GENE EXPRESSION OF PROINFLAMMATORY CYTOKINES, ADHESION MOLECULES NFκB (p50) AND eNOS, IN LPS-STIMULATED HUVECS

IL-6 gene expression (Figure 4.10) was significantly reduced after 16 hours of TEMF (0.3 – 10 μM) and LPS co-incubation in HUVEC scompared to LPS alone ($p < 0.001$). TEMF at lower concentrations (0.3 - 0.6 μM) are the most effective concentration in suppressing the IL-6 gene expression. However, co-incubation of HUVECs with LPS and TEMF (0.3 – 10 μM) did not reduce TNF-α gene expression compared to LPS alone (Figure 4.11).

TEMF at lower concentrations (0.3 - 1.3 μM) but not at higher concentrations (2.5 - 10 μM) significantly suppressed LPS-induced gene expression of ICAM-1 compared to cells incubated with LPS alone ($p < 0.05$) with TEMF at 0.6 μM ($p < 0.01$) being the most potent concentration (Figure 4.12). The incubation of TEMF at all concentrations (0.3 - 10 μM) with LPS significantly reduced the gene expression of VCAM-1 ($p < 0.0001$) compared to LPS alone (Figure 4.13). E-selectin gene expression was reduced in HUVECs co-incubated with LPS plus TEMF across all concentrations (0.3 - 10 μM) compared to LPS alone ($p < 0.05$) (Figure 4.14). The more potent effects were at extremes of the concentration range (i.e 0.3 and 10.0 μM).

47

To define the possible pathway leading to reduce cytokine and adhesion molecules by TEMF, the mRNA expression of NFκB and eNOS were investigated. NFκB gene expression (Figure 4.15) was suppressed by TEMF throughout all concentrations (0.3 - 10 μM) compared to LPS alone in HUVECs (p<0.0001). TEMF at the lower concentrations (0.3 - 1.3 μM) are the most effective concentration in suppressing the NFκB gene expression. There was a trend of increased eNOS gene expression (Figure 4.16) with the co-incubation of LPS and TEMF (0.3 - 10 μM) in HUVECs compared to controls but these did not reach statistical significant levels.

FIGURE 4.9 (a):

Effects of TEMF (0.3 - 10 μM) on the eNOS Protein Expression in LPS Stimulated HUVECs. Prior to Incubation, Cells Lysates Were Obtained and Proceeded With eNOS Immunoassay kit. Results are Expressed as eNOS Concentration (pg/ml). Data are Expressed as Mean ± SD (n=3). * p<0.05, ** p<0.01 and **** p< 0.0001 Compared to HUVECs Incubated With LPS Alone

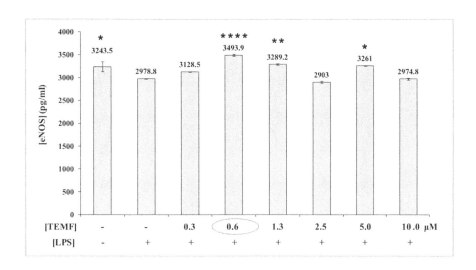

FIGURE 4.9 (b):

% Increment of eNOS by Various Concentrations of TEMF (0.3 – 10 μM) over LPS Stimulated HUVECs. Varying Concentrations of TEMF Were Added to the HUVECSs Together With LPS (1 μg/ml) and Incubated in a Humidified Incubator Set at 37 °C and 5 % CO_2 for 16 Hours. Data Are Expressed as Mean ± SD (n=3). ANOVA p<0.0001

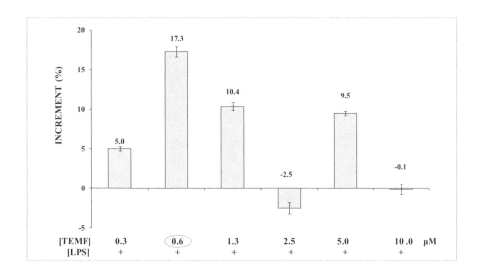

FIGURE 4.10

Effects of TEMF (0.3 - 10 µM) on the IL-6 Gene Expression in LPS Stimulated HUVECs. Prior to Incubation, Total RNA Was Extracted from the Cells and Subjected to Quantitative Real - Time PCR (qPCR) to Determine the IL-6 Gene Expression. Data are Expressed as Mean ± SD (n=3). ** p< 0.01 compared to HUVECs incubated with LPS alone.

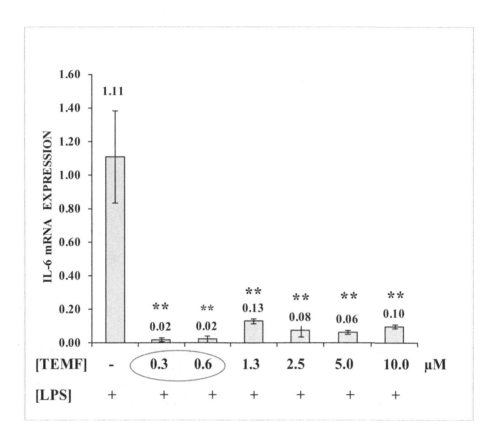

FIGURE 4.11

Effects of TEMF (0.3 - 10 µM) on the TNF-α Gene Expression in LPS Stimulated HUVECs. Prior to Incubation, Total RNA Was Extracted From the Cells and Subjected to Quantitative Real - Time PCR (qPCR) to Determine the TNF-α Gene Expression. Data are Expressed as Mean ± SD (n=3). ** p< 0.01 Compared to HUVECs Incubated With LPS Alone.

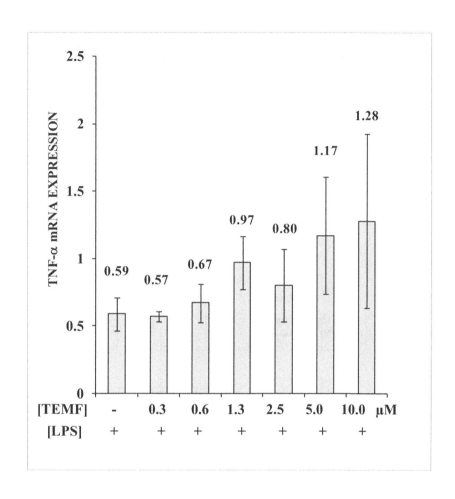

FIGURE 4.12

Effects of TEMF (0.3 – 10 µM) on the ICAM-1 Gene Expression in LPS Stimulated
Cultured HUVECs. Prior to Incubation, Total RNA Was Extracted from the Cells and
Subjected to Quantitative Real - Time PCR (qPCR) to Determine the ICAM-1 Gene
Expression. Data are Expressed as Mean $\pm$ SD (n=3). * p<0.05 and ** p< 0.01
Compared to HUVECs Incubated With LPS Alone

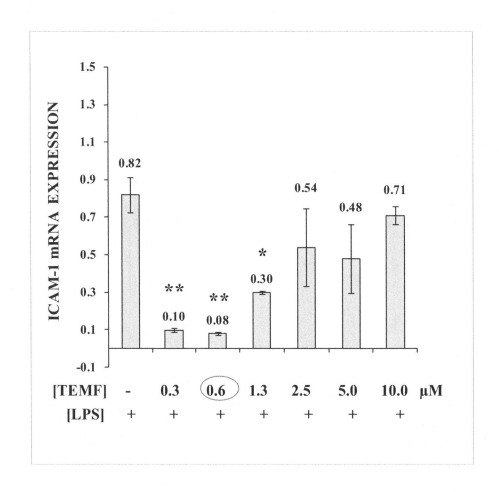

FIGURE 4.13

Effects of TEMF (0.3 – 10 µM) on the VCAM-1 Gene Expression in LPS Stimulated Cultured HUVECs. Prior to Incubation, Total RNA Was Extracted From the Cells and Subjected to Quantitative Real - Time PCR (qPCR) to Determine the VCAM-1 Gene Expression. Data are Expressed as Mean ± SD (n=3). **** p< 0.0001 Compared to HUVECs Incubated With LPS Alone

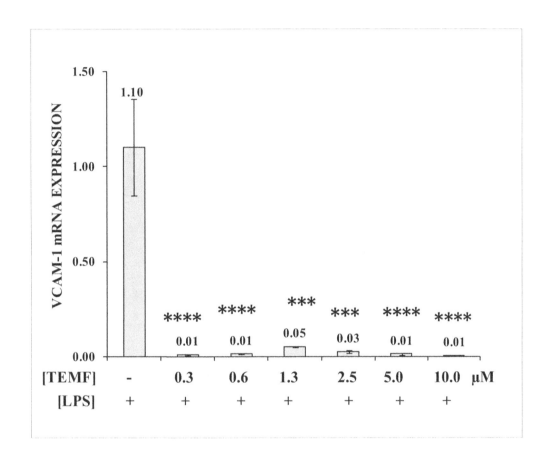

FIGURE 4.14

Effects of TEMF (0.3 – 10 µM) on the e-selectin Gene Expression in LPS Stimulated Cultured HUVECs. Prior to Incubation, Total RNA Was Extracted From the Cells and Subjected to Quantitative Real - Time PCR (qPCR) to Determine E-selectin Gene Expression. Data are Expressed as Mean ± SD (n=3). * p< 0.05 and **p< 0.01 Compared to HUVECs Incubated With LPS Alone

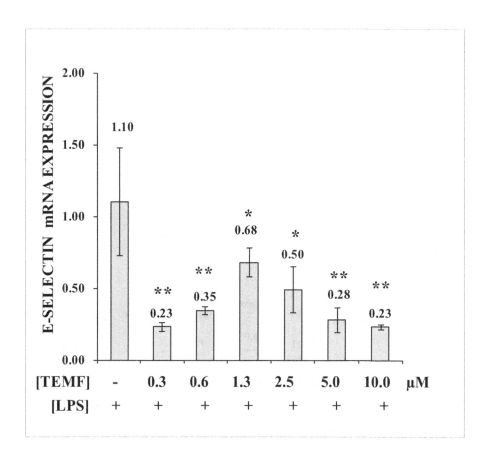

FIGURE 4.15

Effects of TEMF (0.3 – 10 μM) on the NFκB Gene Expression in LPS Stimulated
Cultured HUVECs. Prior to Incubation, Total RNA Was Extracted from the Cells and
Subjected to Quantitative Real - Time PCR (qPCR) to Determine NFκB Gene
Expression. Data are Expressed as Mean ± SD (n=3). **** p< 0.01 Compared to
HUVECs Incubated with LPS alone

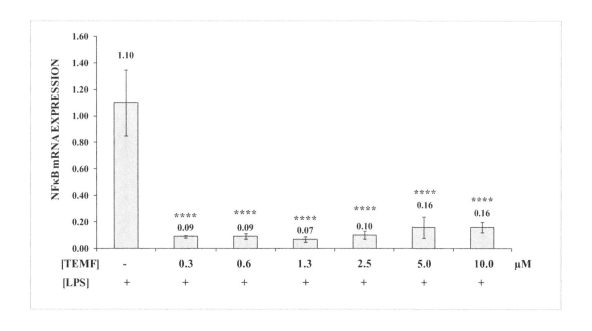

FIGURE 4.16

Effects of TEMF (0.3 – 10 μM) on the eNOS Gene Expression in LPS Stimulated Cultured HUVECs. Prior to Incubation, Total RNA Was Extracted from the cells and Subjected to Quantitative Real- Time PCR (qPCR) to Determine eNOS Gene Expression. Data are Expressed as Mean ± SD (n=3)

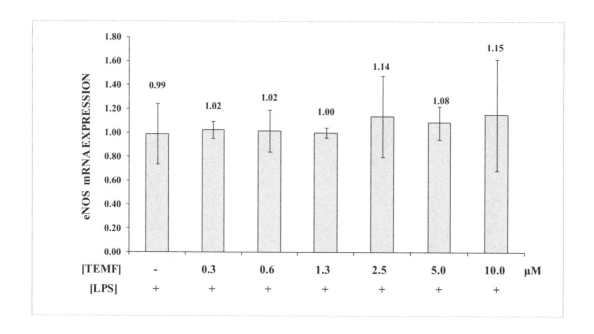

4.7 EFFECTS OF TCT ISOMERS AND α-TOC ON IL-6 PROTEIN SECRETION

TEMF contain a rich fraction of TCT isomers (α-, β-, γ-, δ- TCT) and small amount of α-TOC with TCT: TOC = 2:1 ratio (65.5g: 34.5g). Therefore, the effects of each α-, β-, γ-, δ-TCT isomers and α-TOC on inflammation, endothelial activation and monocytes binding were further investigated. This is important to determine which component of vitamin E in TEMF is responsible for its suppressive effects. The effects of TCT isomers and α-TOC on the secretion of IL-6 in LPS stimulated HUVECs are illustrated in Figure 4.17. Co-incubation of LPS with γ-TCT and δ-

TCT across all concentrations (0.3 μM – 10 μM) reduce the IL-6 secretion (p<0.0001, ANOVA) in HUVECs. α-TCT at 10 μM concentration had a significantly lower production of IL-6 compared to LPS stimulated HUVECs (66.5 ± 1.1 % vs. 100.0 ± 0.0 %, p<0.0001). Similarly, β-TCT at 10 μM concentration significantly reduces the secretion of IL-6 when compared to LPS controls (80.0 ± 0.8 % vs. 100.0 ± 0.0, p<0.05). However, at some concentrations (0.6, 1.3 μM for α-TCT and 2.5, 5.0 μM for β-TCT) IL-6 production was enhanced compared to controls. γ-TCT across all concentrations (0.3 μM – 10 μM) had lower IL-6 production of compared to LPS controls (67.3 ± 0.9 % - 94.7 ± 0.6 % vs. 100.0 ± 0.0 %, p<0.0001 – p<0.05). Production of IL-6 are significantly reduced by δ-TCT at all concentrations (0.3 μM – 10 μM) compared to LPS stimulated HUVECs (71.6 ± 0.3 % - 84.5 ± 3.0 %, p<0.0001 – p<0.05). No statistically significant difference in the production of IL-6 was found between α-TOC at all concentrations (0.3 μM – 10 μM) and LPS controls.

4.8 EFFECTS OF TCT ISOMERS AND α-TOC ON TNF-α PROTEIN SECRETION

The effects of TCT isomers and α-TOC on TNF-α protein secretion was investigated in LPS stimulated HUVECs as illustrated in Figure 4.18. TNF-α protein secretion was unaffected by the co-incubation of TCT isomers or α-TOC with LPS across all concentrations (0.3 μM – 10 μM).

FIGURE 4.17

Effects of TCT Isomers and α-TOC (0.3 μM – 10 μM) on the IL-6 Protein Expression in LPS Stimulated HUVECs. Prior to Incubation, IL-6 Protein Expression in the Supernatant Was Measured by ELISA. Results are Expressed as Percentage (%) of LPS Controls. Data are Expressed as Mean ± SD (n=3). * p<0.05 and **** p< 0.0001 Compared to HUVECs Incubated With LPS Alone

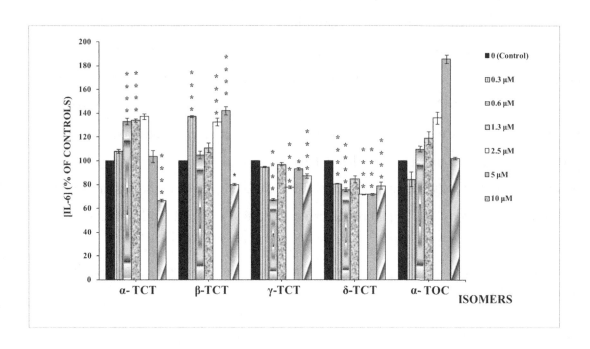

FIGURE 4.18

Effects of TCT isomers and α-TOC (0.3 µM – 10 µM) on the TNF-α Protein Expression in LPS Stimulated HUVECs. Prior to Incubation, TNF-α Protein Expression in the Supernatant was Measured by ELISA. Results are Expressed as Percentage (%) of LPS Controls. Data are Expressed as Mean ± SD (n=3)

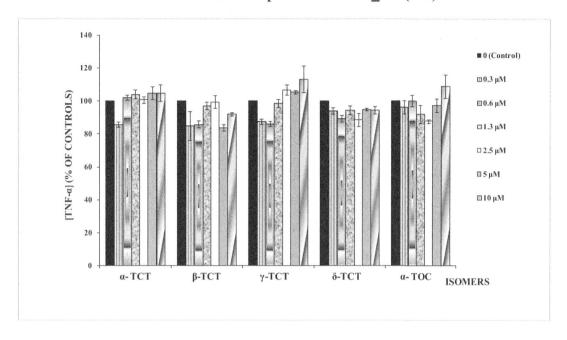

4.9 EFFECTS OF TCT ISOMERS AND α-TOC ON ICAM-1 PROTEIN SECRETION

The effects of TCT isomers and α-TOC on the secretion of ICAM-1 in LPS stimulated HUVECs are illustrated in Figure 4.19. At concentrations 0.3 μM–10 μM, ICAM-1 protein expression was significantly suppressed by all α-, β-, γ- and δ-TCT isomers ($p < 0.0001$, ANOVA) but not by α-TOC in LPS-stimulated HUVECs. In-comparison to LPS alone, co-incubation of LPS with α-TCT at concentrations of 0.3 μM – 10 μM significantly blocked the ICAM-1 protein secretion in HUVECs (49.0 $\pm$ 0.8 % - 68.6 $\pm$ 1.5 % vs. 100.0 $\pm$ 0.0 %, $p < 0.0001$-$p < 0.05$). Similarly, each β-TCT concentration (0.3 μM – 10 μM) had lower production of ICAM-1 than LPS controls (67.7 $\pm$ 1.9 % - 97.4 $\pm$ 3.2 % vs. 100.0 $\pm$ 0.0 %, $p < 0.0001$ - $p < 0.05$) but the potency is less than α-TCT. Co-incubation of LPS and γ-TCT at 0.3 – 10 μM even lead to greater reduction in ICAM-1 protein expression compared to LPS alone (41.7 $\pm$ 1.7 % - 77.5 $\pm$ 1.4 % vs. 100.0 $\pm$ 0.0 %, $p < 0.0001$ - $p < 0.05$). However, the greatest potency of ICAM-1 suppression was showed by δ-TCT at 0.3 – 10 μM concentrations co-incubated with LPS compared to LPS alone (18.8 $\pm$ 0.1 % - 77.5 $\pm$ 5.9 % vs. 100.0 $\pm$ 0.0 %, $p < 0.0001$ - $p < 0.05$). There was no difference ($p > 0.05$) in ICAM-1 production between co-incubation of LPS with α-TOC (0.3 μM – 10 μM) and LPS controls in HUVECs.

4.10 EFFECTS OF TCT ISOMERS AND α-TOC ON VCAM-1 PROTEIN SECRETION

Figure 4.20 illustrates the effects of TCT isomers and α-TOC on VCAM-1 protein secretion in LPS stimulated HUVECs. VCAM-1 production was significantly decreased by γ-TCT and δ-TCT at all concentrations (0.3 μM – 10 μM, $p < 0.0001$, ANOVA). In-comparison to LPS alone, co-incubation of LPS and γ-TCT at concentrations of 0.3 μM – 10 μM significantly blocked the VCAM-1 protein secretion in HUVECs (35.1 $\pm$ 3.7 % - 57.1 $\pm$ 5.4 % vs. 100.0 $\pm$ 0.0 %, $p < 0.0001$). Each δ-TCT concentration (0.3 μM – 10 μM) had lower production of VCAM-1 than LPS controls (26.9 $\pm$ 3.9 % - 62.0 $\pm$ 0.3 % vs. 100.0 $\pm$ 0.0 %, $p < 0.0001$ - $p < 0.01$).

There was no significant VCAM-1 reduction by α-TCT, β-TCT and α-TOC on the production of VCAM-1 in LPS-stimulated HUVECs.

FIGURE 4.19

Effects of TCT Isomers and α-TOC (0.3 μM – 10 μM) on the sICAM-1 Protein Expression in LPS Stimulated HUVECs. Prior to Incubation, sICAM-1 Protein Expression in the Supernatant Was Measured by ELISA. Results are Expressed as Percentage (%) of LPS Controls. Data are Expressed as Mean ± SD (n=3). * p<0.05, ** p<0.01 and **** p< 0.0001 Compared to HUVECs Incubated With LPS Alone.

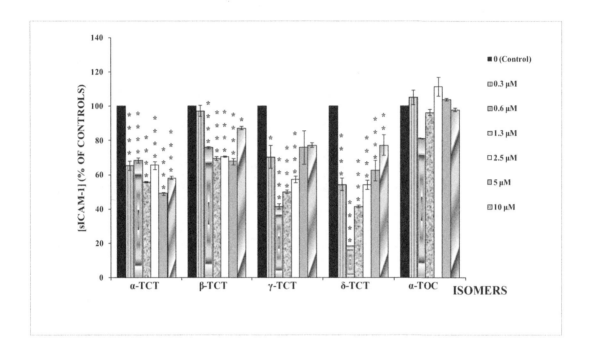

FIGURE 4.20

Effects of TCT Isomers and α-TOC (0.3 μM – 10 μM) on the sVCAM-1 Protein Expression in LPS Stimulated HUVECs. Prior to Incubation, sVCAM-1 Protein Expression in the Supernatant was Measured by ELISA. Results are Expressed as Percentage (%) of LPS Controls. Data are Expressed as Mean ± SD (n=3). * p<0.05, ** p<0.01, *** p<0.001 and **** p< 0.0001 Compared to HUVECs Incubated With LPS Alone

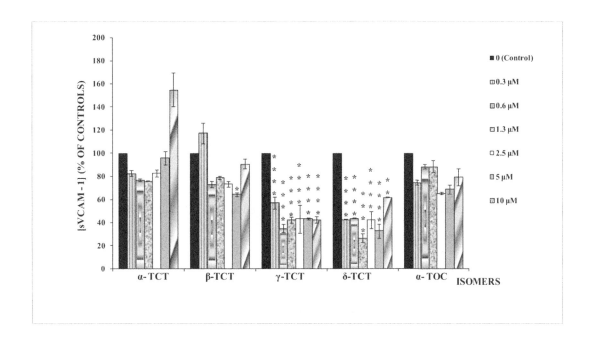

4.11 EFFECTS OF TCT ISOMERS AND α-TOC ON E-SELECTIN PROTEIN SECRETION

Figure 4.21 shows the effects of TCT isomers and α-TOC on e-selectin protein expression in LPS stimulated HUVECs. E-selectin expression was significantly decreased by γ-TCT and δ-TCT across all concentrations in LPS stimulated HUVECs (0.3 μM – 10 μM, p<0.0001, ANOVA). In-comparison to LPS alone, co-incubation of LPS and γ-TCT at concentrations of 0.3 μM – 10 μM significantly blocked the e-selectin protein secretion in HUVECs (42.9 ± 0.4 % - 82.5 ± 3.5 % vs. 100.0 ± 0.0 %, p<0.0001 - p<0.05).   Production of e-selectin was significantly reduced by co-incubation of LPS together with δ-TCT at all concentrations (0.3 μM – 10 μM) compared to LPS alone (20.9 ± 0.6 % - 95.8 ± 4.4 % vs. 100.0 ± 0.0 %, p<0.0001 - p<0.05). There was no significant reduction of e-selectin production in LPS stimulated HUVECs compared to controls with α-TCT, β-TCT and α-TOC. It is noted that at high concentrations of 10 μM, both α- and β-TCT lead to higher e-selectin production compared to controls (α- TCT: 125.7 ± 8.3 % vs. 100.0 ± 0.0 %, p<0.05; β- TCT: 135.9 ± 6.1 % vs. 100.0 ± 0.0 %, p<0.01).

4.12 EFFECTS OF TCT ISOMERS AND α-TOC ON MONOCYTES BINDING ACTIVITY IN LPS-STIMULATED HUVECs

The effects of TCT isomers and α-TOC on the secretion of monocytes binding activity in LPS stimulated HUVECs are illustrated in Figure 4.22. It was found that α-, β-, γ-, δ- TCT (p<0.0001) but not α-TOC throughout all concentrations lead to reduction of monocytes binding activity. For α- TCT, significant reduction of monocytes binding activity was only observed at 1.3 μM concentration compared to LPS stimulated HUVECs (64.2 ± 5.8 % vs. 100.0 ± 0.0 %, p<0.01). At the concentrations of 0.3 μM – 10 μM, the monocytes binding activity was significantly reduced by β- TCT (53.0 ± 5.3 % – 76.8 ± 10.0 % vs. 100.0 ± 0.0 %, p<0.0001-p<0.001), γ-TCT (54.4 ± 2.9 % - 79.7 ± 13.8 % vs. 100.0 ± 0.0 %, p<0.0001) and δ-TCT (47.6 ± 5.9 % - 68.8 ± 3.9 % vs. 100.0 ± 0.0 %, p<0.0001) in comparison to LPS stimulated HUVECs. In contrast, α-TOC at 0.3 μM (197.9 ± 3.7 % vs. 100.0 ± 0.0 %, p<0.0001) and 5 μM (111.1 ± 19.6 % vs. 100.0 ± 0.0 %, p<0.01) showed a significant increment on monocytes binding activity compared to LPS stimulated HUVECs.

FIGURE 4.21

Effects of TCT Isomers and α-TOC (0.3 μM – 10 μM) on the E-Selectin Protein Expression in LPS Stimulated HUVECs. Prior to Incubation, E-selectin Protein Expression in the Supernatant Was Measured by ELISA. Results are Expressed as Percentage (%) of LPS Controls. Data are Expressed as Mean ± SD (n=3).   * p<0.05, ** p<0.01 and **** p< 0.0001 Compared to HUVECs Incubated with LPS Alone

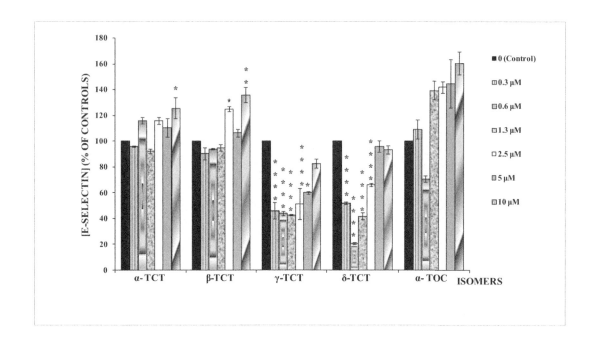

FIGURE 4.22

Effects of TCT Isomers and α-TOC (0.3 μM – 10 μM) on the Monocytes Binding Activity in LPS Stimulated Cultured HUVECs. Prior to Incubation, Cells Were Subjected to the Monocytes Binding Assay. Results are Expressed as Percentage (%) of LPS Controls. Data are Expressed as Mean ± SD (n=3). * p<0.05, ** p<0.01, *** p<0.001 and **** p< 0.0001 Compared to HUVECs Incubated With LPS Alone

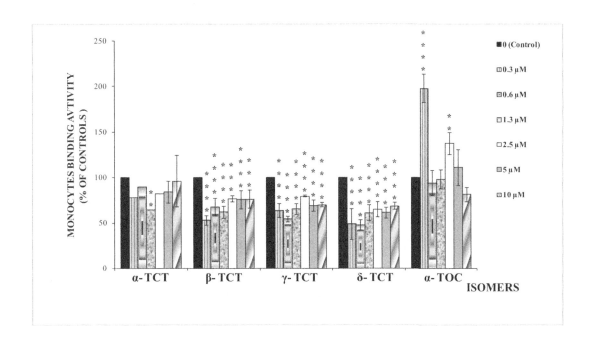

4.13 EFFECTS OF TCT ISOMERS AND α-TOC ON NFκB BINDING ACTIVITY IN LPS-STIMULATED HUVECs

LPS mediated the activation of NFκB through enhancing the phosphorylation, ubiquination and proteolytic degradation of IκB. This processes lead to the translocation of NFκB into the nucleus. The free NFκB in nucleus can activate the expression of cytokines and adhesion molecules and facilitate the migration of monocytes into the tunica intima, the key event in the pathogenesis of atherosclerosis. Figure 4.23 shows the effects of TCT isomers and α-TOC on NFκB binding activity in LPS stimulated HUVEC. Co-incubation of LPS and α-, β-, γ-, δ-TCT across all concentrations (0.3 μM – 10 μM) reduced the NFκB binding activity ($p < 0.0001$, ANOVA) in HUVECs. On the other hand, α- TOC has no effect on NFκB binding activity in LPS stimulated HUVECs. Most concentrations of α-TCT except for 0.6 μM significantly reduced the NFκB binding activity when compared to untreated LPS-stimulated controls. (79.4 $\pm$ 0.2 % - 88.9 $\pm$ 0.4 vs. 100.0 $\pm$ 0.0, $p < 0.0001$ - $p < 0.01$) No statistically significant difference in NFκB binding activity was found between β- TCT at all concentrations (0.3 μM – 10 μM) and LPS controls. In contrast, there was a significant reduction of NFκB binding activity by γ- TCT (76.5 $\pm$ 1.9 % - 81.3 $\pm$ 2.8 %, $p < 0.0001$ and δ- TCT (76.0 $\pm$ 2.8 % - 84.0 $\pm$ 2.9 %, $p < 0.0001$ – $p < 0.01$). Similarly, δ-TCT across all concentration (0.3 μM – 10 μM), reduces NFκB binding activity ($p < 0.0001$-$p < 0.01$). There was no reduction in NFκB activation in LPS stimulated HUVECs co-incubated with α- TOC compared to LPS controls across all concentrations (0.3 μM – 10 μM).

4.14 EFFECTS OF TCT ISOMERS AND α-TOC ON ENOS SECRETION IN LPS-STIMULATED HUVECs

Figure 4.24 shows the effects of TCT isomers and α- TOC on eNOS secretion in LPS stimulated HUVECs. There was no beneficial effect in terms of increment of eNOS production by α- TCT, β- TCT and α- TOC in LPS stimulated HUVECs. There was a significant increment of eNOS production by γ-TCT at the concentrations of 5 μM and 10 μM compared to LPS controls (5 μM: 147.1 $\pm$ 12.4 % vs. 100.0 $\pm$ 0.0 %, $p < 0.01$; 10 μM: 148.2 $\pm$ 3.6 % vs. 100.0 $\pm$ 0.0 %, $p < 0.01$). Co-incubation of LPS and δ-TCT at 1.3 μM and 2.5 μM significantly increased the production of eNOS in HUVECs (1.3 μM: 120.2 ± 0.1 % vs. 100.0 ± 0.0 %, $p<0.05$; 2.5 μM: 117.6 ± 2.0 vs. 100.0 ± 0.0 %, $p<0.01$).

FIGURE 4.23

Effects of TCT Isomers and α-TOC (0.3 μM – 10 μM) on the NFκB Binding Activity in LPS Stimulated Cultured HUVECs. Prior to Incubation, Nuclear Extracts were isolated and the level of NFκB Transcriptional Activation Was Measured by NFκB p50 Transcription Factor Assay kit. Results are Expressed as percentage (%) of LPS controls. Data are Expressed as Mean ± SD (n=3). * p<0.05 and **** p< 0.0001 Compared to HUVECs Incubated with LPS Alone

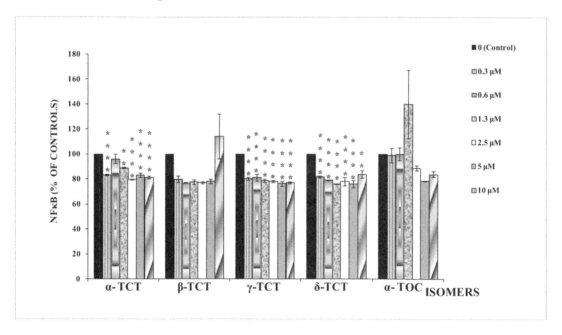

FIGURE 4.24

Effects of TCT Isomers and α-TOC (0.3 µM – 10 µM) on the eNOS Protein in LPS Stimulated Cultured HUVECs. Prior to Incubation, Cells Lysates Were Obtained Proceeded with eNOS Immunoassay kit. Results are Expressed as Percentage (%) of LPS Controls.
Data are Expressed as Mean ± SD (n=3). * p<0.05 and ** p< 0.01 Compared to HUVECs Incubated with LPS Alone

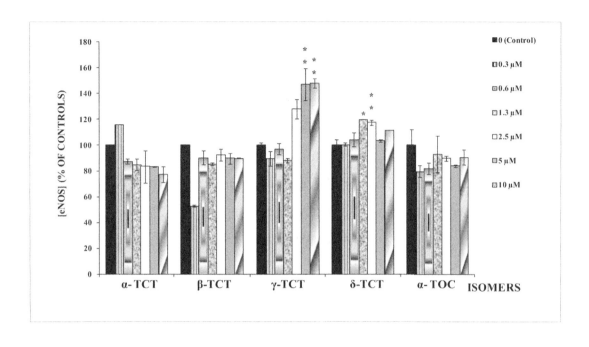

4.15 EFFECTS OF TCT ISOMERS AND α-TOC ON IL-6 GENE EXPRESSION IN LPS-STIMULATED HUVECs

Figure 4.25 illustrates the effects of TCT isomers and α-TOC on IL-6 gene expression in LPS stimulated HUVECs. α- TCT and δ-TCT almost all concentrations (0.3 μM – 10 μM) significantly downregulated the IL-6 mRNA expression in LPS stimulated HUVECs (p<0.0001, ANOVA). In comparison to HUVECs incubated with LPS alone, α-TCT at 0.3 and 1.3 μM downregulated the IL-6 mRNA expression (0.3 μM: 0.17 ± 0.02 vs. 1.00 ± 0.00 fold change, p<0.01; 1.3 μM: 0.23 ± 0.06 vs. 1.00 ± 0.00 fold change, p<0.05). Co-incubation of LPS with β-TCT at 0.6 μM – 10 μM concentrations significantly reduced the gene expression of IL-6 compared the LPS alone (0.54 ± 0.01 –0.93 ± 0.02 vs. 1.0 ± 0.0 fold change, p<0.0001 - p<0.05). Co-incubation of LPS together with γ-TCT at lower concentration (0.3 μM -1.3 μM) significantly reduced the IL-6 mRNA expression compared to LPS alone (0.07 ± 0.00 – 0.31 ± 0.04 vs. 1.00 ± 0.00 fold change, p<0.0001 – p<0.05). However at higher concentrations (2.5 μM – 10 μM), γ- TCT leads to increased IL-6 gene expression compared to LPS controls (1.25 ± 0.03 – 1.79 ± 0.08 fold change, p<0.05). At concentrations of 0.3 μM - 10 μM, δ-TCT suppressed the IL-6 gene expression compared to LPS alone (0.14 ± 0.01 – 0.49 ± 0.07 vs. 1.00 ± 0.00 fold change, p<0.0001). There was an increased trend in IL-6 gene expression with co-incubation of α-TOC (0.3 μM – 10 μM) compared to LPS controls, but this did not reach statistically significant level.

4.16 EFFECTS OF TCT ISOMERS AND α-TOC ON TNF-α GENE EXPRESSION IN LPS-STIMULATED HUVECs

The effects of TCT isomers and α-TOC on TNF-α gene expression was investigated in LPS stimulation HUVECs as illustrated in Figure 4.26. Co-incubation of LPS with γ-TCT at low concentrations (0.3 μM -1.3 μM) downregulated the TNF-α gene expression compared to LPS controls ($0.17 \pm 0.07 - 0.40 \pm 0.17$ vs. 1.00 ± 0.00 fold change, $p<0.0001$ - $p<0.05$). However at higher concentration (5 μM -10 μM) γ-TCT appeared to enhance TNF-α gene expression ($1.92 \pm 0.01 - 2.12 \pm 0.12$ vs. 1.00 ± 0.00 fold change, ($p<0.0001$ - $p<0.01$). Co-incubation with α- TCT, β- TCT, δ- TCT and α- TOC together with LPS had no significant TNF-α reduction compared to LPS controls.

FIGURE 4.25

Effects of TCT Isomers and α-TOC (0.3 μM – 10 μM) on the IL-6 Gene Expression in
LPS Stimulated HUVECs. Prior to Incubation, Total RNA was Extracted from the
Cells and Subjected to Quantitative Real - Time PCR (qPCR) to Determine the IL-6
Gene Expression. Each data was Normalized to 1.0 (HUVECs Incubated with LPS
Alone) and GAPDH Reference Gene. Data are Expressed as Mean ± SD (n=3). *
p<0.05, ** p<0.01 and **** p< 0.0001 Compared to HUVECs Incubated With LPS
Alone

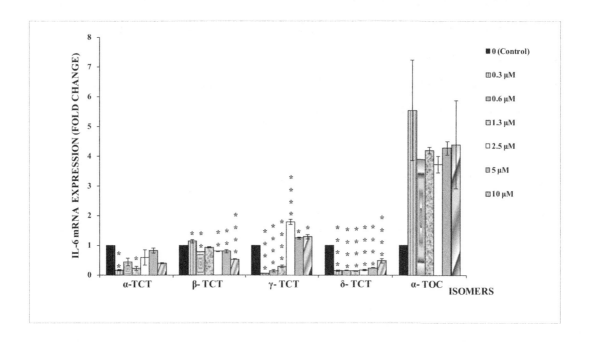

FIGURE 4.26

Effects of TCT Isomers and α-TOC (0.3 μM – 10 μM) on the TNF-α Gene Expression in LPS Stimulated HUVECs. Prior to Incubation, Total RNA was Extracted from the Cells and Subjected to Quantitative Real - Time PCR (qPCR) to Determine the TNF-α Gene Expression. Each data was Normalized to 1.0 (HUVECs Incubated With LPS Alone) and GAPDH Reference Gene. Data are Expressed as Mean ± SD (n=3). * p<0.05, ** p<0.01 and **** p< 0.0001 Compared to HUVECs Incubated with LPS Alone

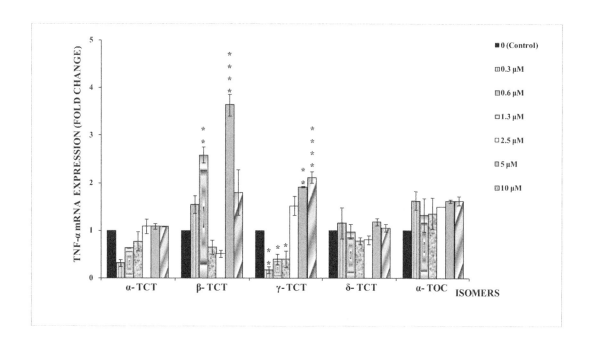

4.17 EFFECTS OF TCT ISOMERS AND α-TOC ON ICAM-1 GENE EXPRESSION IN LPS-STIMULATED HUVECs

Figure 4.27 shows the effects of TCT isomers and α-TOC on ICAM-1 gene expression in LPS stimulated HUVECs. α- and γ-TCT at all concentrations (0.3 μM – 10 μM) downregulated the ICAM-1 mRNA expression in LPS stimulated HUVECs ($p < 0.0001$, ANOVA). In comparison to HUVECs incubated with LPS alone, α-TCT at 0.3 μM - 10 μM suppressed the ICAM-1 mRNA expression ($0.01 \pm 0.00 – 0.55 \pm 0.06$ vs. 1.00 ± 0.00 fold change, $p < 0.0001$). At concentration of 0.3 μM - 10 μM, δ-TCT suppressed the ICAM-1 gene expression compared to LPS-stimulate HUVECs alone ($0.18 \pm 0.01 – 0.35 \pm 0.03$ vs. 1.00 ± 0.00 fold change, $p < 0.0001$). Co-incubation of LPS with β-TCT at 2.5 μM and 5 μM concentrations significantly reduced the gene expression of ICAM-1 compared the LPS alone ($0.45 \pm 0.09 – 0.48 \pm 0.03$ vs. 1.00 ± 0.00 fold change, $p < 0.01 – p < 0.05$). There was a reduced trend of ICAM-1 mRNA expression by co-incubation of γ-TCT with LPS but it did not reach statistical significant level. In contrast, there was a marked increment of ICAM-1 mRNA expression in α- TOC at all concentrations (0.3 μM – 10 μM) compared to LPS controls ($1.99 \pm 0.28 – 2.20 \pm 0.10$ vs. 1.00 ± 0.00 fold change, $p < 0.0001$ - $p < 0.05$).

4.18 EFFECTS OF TCT ISOMERS AND α-TOC ON VCAM-1 GENE EXPRESSION IN LPS-STIMULATED HUVECs

Figure 4.28 shows the effects of TCT isomers and α-TOC on VCAM-1 mRNA expression in LPS stimulated HUVECs. Only δ-TCT at all concentrations (0.3 μM – 10 μM) has profound significant reduction of VCAM-1 mRNA expression in LPS stimulated HUVECs ($p < 0.0001$, ANOVA). Co-incubation of LPS and α- TCT downregulated VCAM-1 mRNA expression compared to LPS alone at 0.3 μM (0.55 ± 0.02 vs. 1.00 ± 0.00 fold change, $p < 0.05$). Co-incubation of LPS with low concentrations of β- TCT (0.3 μM – 1.3 μM) increased the VCAM-1 mRNA expression compared to LPS alone ($1.96 \pm 0.01 – 2.01 \pm 0.06$ vs. 1.00 ± 0.00 fold change, $p < 0.05$) which at higher concentration (2.5 – 10 μM) reduced VCAM-1 gene expression ($0.38 \pm 0.02 - 0.51 \pm 0.03$ vs. $1.00 + 0.00$ fold change, $p<0.01 - p<0.05$). In contrast, co-incubation of LPS together with γ- TCT at lower concentration (0.3 μM - 1.3 μM) significantly suppressed the VCAM-1 mRNA expression compared to LPS alone ($0.01 \pm 0.00 - 0.12 \pm 0.04$ vs. 1.00 ± 0.00 fold change, $p<0.01$ but at higher concentration (2.5 μM - 10 μM) γ-TCT significantly increased the VCAM-1 mRNA expression compared to HUVEC stimulated with LPS alone ($1.7\ 0 \pm 0.07 - 2.10 \pm 0.18$ vs. 1.00 ± 0.00 fold change, $p<0.01$ - $p<0.05$). δ- TCT at all concentrations (0.3 μM – 10.0 μM) co-incubated with LPS showed significant suppressive effect on the VCAM-1 mRNA expression compared to LPS controls ($0.09 \pm 0.01 - 0.13 \pm 0.02$ vs. 1.00 ± 0.00 fold change, $p<0.0001$). No statistically significant difference in VCAM-1 mRNA expression was found between α-TOC (0.3 μM – 10 μM) and LPS controls.

FIGURE 4.27

Effects of TCT Isomers and α-TOC (0.3 μM– 10 μM) on the ICAM-1 Gene eExpression in LPS Stimulated HUVECs. Prior to Incubation, Total RNA was Extracted from the Cells and Subjected to Quantitative Real - Time PCR (qPCR) to Determine the ICAM-1 Gene Expression. Each Data was Normalized to 1.0 (HUVECs Incubated with LPS Alone) and GAPDH Reference Gene. Data are Expressed as Mean ± SD (n=3). * p<0.05, ** p<0.01 and **** p< 0.0001 Compared to HUVECs Incubated with LPS Alone

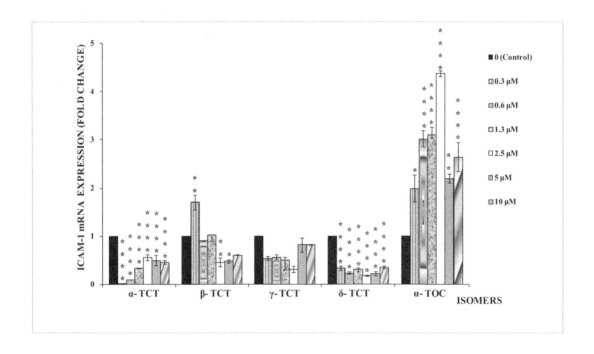

FIGURE 4.28

Effects of TCT Isomers and α-TOC (0.3 μM – 10 μM) on the VCAM-1 Gene Expression in LPS Stimulated Cultured HUVECs. Prior to Incubation, Total RNA was Extracted from the Cells and Subjected to Quantitative Real - Time PCR (qPCR) to Determine the VCAM-1 Gene Expression. Each Data was Normalized to 1.0 (HUVECs Incubated with LPS Alone) and GAPDH Reference Gene. Data are Expressed as Mean ± SD (n=3). * p<0.05, ** p<0.01 and **** p< 0.0001 Compared to HUVECs Incubated with LPS Alone

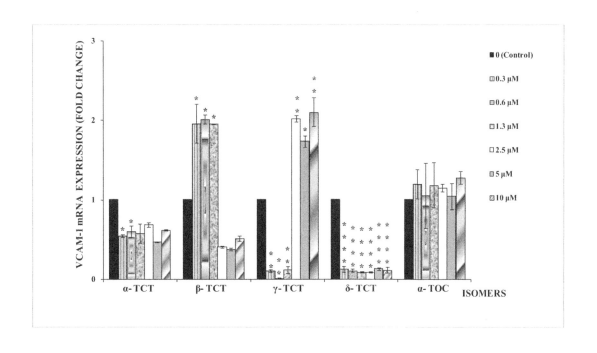

4.19 EFFECTS OF TCT ISOMERS AND α-TOC ON E-SELECTIN GENE EXPRESSION IN LPS-STIMULATED HUVECs

Figure 4.29 illustrates the effects of TCT isomers and α-TOC on e-selectin gene expression in LPS stimulated HUVECs. γ- TCT and δ- TCT across all concentrations (0.3 μM – 10 μM) downregulated the e-selectin mRNA expression in LPS stimulated HUVECs (p<0.0001, ANOVA). There was a reduced trend in the downregulation of e-selectin mRNA expression by co-incubation of α-TCT and LPS but it was not statistically significant when compared to LPS controls alone. In comparison to HUVECs incubated with LPS alone, β- TCT at 1.3-10 μM downregulated the e-selectin mRNA expression (0.22 ± 0.02 – 0.38 ± 0.02 vs. 1.00 ± 0.00 fold change, p<0.01 – p<0.05. Co-incubation of LPS with γ-TCT at 0.3 μM and 0.6 μM concentrations significantly reduced the gene expression of e-selectin compared the LPS alone (0.3 μM: 0.14 ± 0.02 vs. 1.00 ± 0.00 fold change, p<0.01; 0.6 μM: 0.28 ± 0.00 vs. 1.00 ± 0.00 fold change, p<0.01). At concentrations of 0.3 μM - 10 μM, δ-TCT suppressed the e-selectin gene expression compared to LPS alone (0.18 ± 0.01 – 0.49 ± 0.02 vs. 1.00 ± 0.00 fold change, p<0.0001). There was no statistically significant difference in e-selectin mRNA expression was found between α-TOC (0.3 μM – 10 μM) and LPS controls.

4.20 EFFECTS OF TCT ISOMERS AND α-TOC ON NFκB GENE EXPRESSION IN LPS-STIMULATED HUVECs

Figure 4.30 shows the effects of TCT isomers and α-TOC on NFκB gene expression in LPS stimulated HUVECs. δ-TCT at 0.3 μM – 5.0 μM co-incubated with LPS showed significant suppressive effect on the NFκB gene expression compared to LPS controls (0.25 ± 0.04 – 0.43 ± 0.00 vs. 1.00 ± 0.00 fold change, p<0.01 - p< 0.0001). In-comparison to LPS alone, co-incubation of LPS and α-TCT at lower concentrations (0.3 - 0.6 μM) significantly blocked the NFκB gene expression (0.3 μM: 0.07 ± 0.00 vs. 1.00 ± 0.00 fold change, p<0.0001; 0.6 μM: 0.14 ± 0.01 vs. 1.00 ± 0.00 fold change, p<0.0001). Co-incubation of LPS together with γ-TCT at low concentrations (0.3 μM - 1.3 μM) significantly blocked the NFκB expression compared to LPS alone (0.03 ± 0.01– 0.08 ± 0.10 fold change, $p<0.0001$). However both α- and γ- TCT at higher concentrations did not lead to reduce NFκB gene expression. In contrast, co-incubation of LPS with β- TCT at higher concentrations (5 μM -10 μM) lead to reduce NFκB gene expression compared to LPS alone (5 μM: 0.56 ± 0.03 vs. 1.00 ± 0.00 fold change, $p<0.0001$; 10 μM: 0.37 ± 0.04 vs. 1.00 ± 0.00 fold change , $p<0.0001$) but not do so at lower concentration (0.3 μM – 2.5 μM). Co-incubation of LPS and α-TOC at almost all concentrations leading to increase NFκB gene expression compared to LPS alone (1.12 ± 0.01 – 2.77 ± 0.05 vs. 1.00 ± 0.00 fold change, $p<0.01$ - $p<0.0001$).

FIGURE 4.29

Effects of TCT Isomers and α-TOC (0.3 μM – 10 μM) on the e-selectin Gene Expression in LPS Stimulated HUVECs. Prior to Incubation, Total RNA Was extracted from the Cells and subjected to Quantitative Real - Time PCR (qPCR) to determine the E-selectin Gene Expression. Each Data was Normalized to 1.0 (HUVECs incubated with LPS alone) and GAPDH Reference Gene. Data are Expressed as Mean ± SD (n=3). * $p < 0.05$, ** $p < 0.01$ and **** $p < 0.0001$ Compared to HUVECs Incubated with LPS Alone

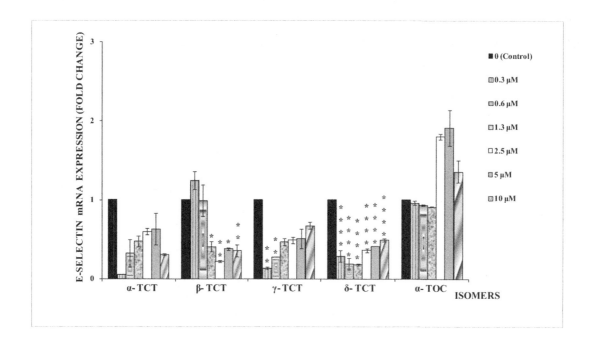

FIGURE 4.30

Effects of TCT Isomers and α-TOC (0.3 μM – 10 μM) on the NFκB Gene Expression in
LPS Stimulated HUVECs. Prior to Incubation, Total RNA was Extracted from the
Cells and Subjected to Quantitative Real - Time PCR (qPCR) to Determine the NFκB
Gene Expression. Each Data was Normalized to 1.0 (HUVECs Incubated with LPS
Alone) and GAPDH Reference Gene. Data are Expressed as Mean $\pm$ SD (n=3).
** p<0.01 and **** p<0.0001 Compared to HUVECs Incubated with LPS Alone

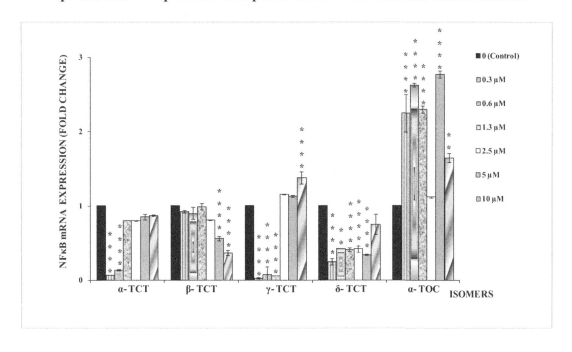

83

4.21 EFFECTS OF TCT ISOMERS AND α-TOC ON eNOS GENE EXPRESSION IN LPS-STIMULATED HUVECs

Figure 4.31 shows the effects of TCT isomers and α-TOC on eNOS gene expression in LPS stimulated HUVECs. There was no beneficial effect in terms of increment of eNOS gene expression by α-TCT co-incubated with LPS compared to LPS alone. There was a significant increment of eNOS gene expression by β- TCT at the concentrations of 0.3 μM - 0.6 μM (0.30 ± 0.00 - 0.89 ± 0.01 vs. $1.00 + 0.00$ fold change, $p<0.01 - p<0.0001$) and 5 μM - 10 μM ($1.60 \pm 0.00 - 1.76 \pm 0.04$ vs. 1.00 ± 0.00 fold change, $p<0.01$) compared to LPS controls. Co-incubation of LPS and γ- TCT at 2.5 μM – 10 μM showed a greater increment of eNOS gene expression compared to LPS alone ($8.28 \pm 0.08 – 11.09 \pm 0.00$ vs. 1.00 ± 0.00 fold change, $p<0.0001$). There was an increased trend in the upregulation of eNOS gene expression by co-incubation of δ- TCT and LPS but it was not statistically significant when compared to LPS controls. Co-incubation of LPS and α- TOC at 5 μM showed a slightly increased in eNOS gene expression compared to LPS controls (1.57 ± 0.05 vs. 1.00 ± 0.00 fold change, $p<0.05$).

FIGURE 4.31

Effects of TCT Isomers and α-TOC (0.3 μM – 10 μM) on the eNOS Gene Expression in LPS Stimulated Cultured HUVECs. Prior to Incubation, Total RNA was Extracted from the Cells and Subjected to Quantitative Real - Time PCR (qPCR) to Determine the eNOS Gene Xxpression. Each Data was Normalized to 1.0 (HUVECs Incubated with LPS Alone) and GAPDH Reference Gene. Data are expressed as Mean ± SD (n=3). * p<0.05, ** p<0.01 and **** p< 0.0001 Compared to HUVECs Incubated with LPS Alone

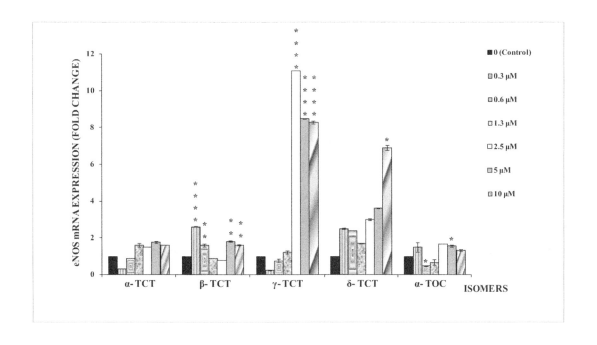

4.22 DETERMINATION OF THE MOST POTENT TCT ISOMERS

To determine the most potent TCT isomers, the analysis of area under the curve (AUC) for each TCT isomers, α-TOC and TEMF for all concentrations combined (0.3 μM – 10 μM) was performed using the Graph Version 4.3 software. After obtaining the AUC for each TCT isomers, α-TOC and TEMF, the percentage (%) inhibition against their respective controls were calculated for each biomarker and illustrated in Table 4.1. δ- TCT shows the highest percentage inhibition of IL-6, ICAM-1 and VCAM-1 protein and gene expression compared to α-TCT, β-TCT, γ-TCT and α-TOC in LPS-stimulated HUVECs. The highest inhibition of monocytes binding activity in LPS stimulated HUVECs was shown by δ-TCT compared to α-TCT, β- TCT, γ- TCT and α- TOC. Furthermore, δ-TCT gives maximum percentage inhibition of NFκB activation compared to α- TCT, β- TCT, γ- TCT and α- TOC in LPS-stimulated HUVECs. For e-selectin protein expression, the highest percentage inhibition was shown by γ- TCT, where as e-selectin gene expression was maximally inhibited by δ- TCT isomer. The highest increment of eNOS protein and gene expression was shown by γ- TCT compared to α- TCT, β- TCT, δ- TCT and α- TOC in LPS stimulated HUVECs. α-TOC significantly increases IL-6 and e-selectin protein expression and monocyte binding activity. α-TOC did not reduce TNF-α, ICAM-1 and VCAM-1 protein expression. In addition, α-TOC did not suppress NFκB activation. α-TOC did not induce eNOS protein expression in LPS stimulated HUVECs. In addition, α-TOC induces ICAM-1 and NFκB gene expression. There was an increased trend of IL-6, VCAM-1 and e-selectin gene expression by α-TOC in LPS stimulated HUVECs. α-TOC did not increase eNOS gene expression. Pure TCT particularly γ- and δ- isomers clearly exhibited to have greater potency than TEMF by showing greater reduction of IL6, ICAM-1, VCAM-1, NFκB and monocyte binding activity (MBA). In addition, γ- and δ TCT isomers have greater potency than TEMF in inducing eNOS expression in LPS stimulated HUVECs. This enhances observation that pure TCT isomers have beneficial effects in terms of inflammation and endothelial activation and α- TOC have detrimental effects to TCT benefits. TCT in combination with α-TOC still have the goodies but inferior to that pure TCT particularly γ- and δ- isomers.

TABLE 4.1

	IL-6 % INHIBIT		TNF-α % INHIBIT		ICAM-1 % INHIBIT		VCAM-1 % INHIBIT		E-SEL % INHIBIT		MBA % INHIBIT	NFκB % INHIBIT		eNOS % INCREMENT	
	P	G	P	G	P	G	P	G	P	G		P	G	P	G
α-TCT	-8.2	36.1	-7.8	-8.2	37.0	50.5	-7.8	43.3	-15.4	44.3	15.9	17.3	28.4	19.2	-69.1
β-TCT	-22.5	24.7	8.7	-114.4	28.2	48.5	27.8	45.4	-17.9	64.9	24.5	16.0	37.7	8.3	-35.1
γ-TCT	12.0	-33.0	-7.4	-74.2	31.7	34.0	57.6	-76.3	38.4	45.4	28.1	22.2	-10.3	-37.5	-757.7
δ-TCT	25.6	73.2	6.9	-1.0	38.8	76.3	59.3	88.7	17.7	60.8	35.7	22.4	53.6	-11.2	-296.9
α-TOC	-50.4	- 309.3	3.2	-55.7	-3.7	-199.0	27.5	-13.4	-47.6	-68.0	-6.3	10.9	-106.2	11.8	43.3
TEMF (2:1)	0.94	92.8	-3.8	-85.4	29.4	34.1	22.44	97.9	52.5	66.0	20.5	15.6	87.6	-4.6	-11.8

% Inhibition of Inflammation and Endothelial Activation Biomarkers, Monocytes Binding activity, NFκB and eNOS by TCT Isomers, α-TOC and TEMF Based on Area Under the Curve Analysis % - Percentage, INHIBIT- Inhibition, P-Protein, G-gene, TCT- Tocotrienol, TOC-Tocopherol & TEMF – Tocotrienol Enriched Mixed Fraction

CHAPTER FIVE
DISCUSSION

5.1   EFFECTS OF TEMF ON MONOCYTES BINDING ACTIVITY, INFLAMMATION AND ENDOTHELIAL ACTIVATION IN ENDOTHELIAL CELLS

In this study, it has been found out that LPS stimulation of HUVECs enhanced the endothelial cell production of IL-6, TNF-α, sICAM-1, sVCAM-1 and e-selectin, NFκB and reduces eNOS expression at the gene and protein levels. LPS activates the canonical/classical pathway leading to the activation of the IκB kinase (IKK). Activation of IKK complex results in phosphorylation of IκB followed by the polyubiquitination and degradation by the proteosome and release of NFκB (Chen, 2005). The free NFκB translocates to the nucleus where it binds to the specific gene promoters and initiates transcription of target genes including pro-inflammatory cytokines and cell adhesion molecules (Chen, 2005).   NFκB p50 is one of the subunits of NFκB family that plays a crucial role in atherosclerosis (Kanters et al., 2004).   Deletion of NFκB1 p50 receptors in mice caused a significant reduction in lesion size and IL-6 (Kanters et al., 2004).   It has been reported that p50 subunits are present in the nucleus of human atherosclerotic plaque cells (Monaco et al., 2004). NFκB p50 is generated by the proteolytic cleavage of precursor protein p105 which is coded by the NFκB1 gene (Kanters et al., 2004).   NFκB1 p50 binds to the kappa-B consensus sequence, located in the enhancer region of genes, which are involved in acute phase reactions (Martinez et al., 2012). Targeting proteins that control the NF-κB signalling pathway regulating the proteolysis of p105 may be useful for treatment of inflammatory diseases (Bienke & Ley, 2004). It has been suggested that any supplement or treatment that are able to deactivate NFκB transcriptional factor can thus inhibit these pro-inflammatory cytokines and adhesion molecules which in turn will be capable of slowing down the progression of atherosclerosis. (Theriault et al., 2002)

To ensure that the observed inhibition of the inflammatory and endothelial activation biomarkers produced by the endothelial cells was not a false positive due to cytotoxic effects, cells viability assay was performed. This assay showed that the cell viability was unaffected up to TEMF concentration of 10 μM. Hence, in this study, the effects of TEMF, pure TCT isomers and α-TOC were examined at concentrations between 0.3 - 10 μM.

This present study showed that co-incubation of LPS stimulated HUVECs with TEMF effectively inhibit the protein and gene expression of IL-6, sICAM-1, sVCAM-1, e-selectin, monocytes binding activity and NFκB p50 activation. TEMF also leads to increased eNOS protein and gene expression. These findings suggest that reduction of monocytes binding activity by TEMF is attributed to the decreased IL-6 and adhesion molecules. In this study, it has been also shown that the reduction of IL-6 and adhesion molecules is through the ability of TEMF in inhibiting the NFκB activation in human endothelial cells. To our knowledge this is the first *in vitro* study to describe the effects of TCTs in each step of atherosclerosis starting from inflammation till monocytes adherence to the endothelial cells. This present study also adds knowledge enhancement potential anti-atherogenic property of TCT which has scarcity of published data.

To date, the ability of TEMF in reducing IL-6 was reported in the macrophages and monocytes cells but none has been studied endothelial cells. Several researchers have found that TEMF at 5 - 30 μg/ml significantly suppressed IL-6 production in macrophages and monocytes cells (Ng & Ko, 2012; Yam at al., 2009; Wu et al., 2008). Similarly, this present study reported the ability of TEMF in reducing IL-6 protein and gene expression in human endothelial cells even at a much lower concentration (0.2 μg/ml = 0.3 μM).

In contrast, this study demonstrated that TEMF did not show beneficial effects in the reduction of protein and gene expression of TNF-α in human endothelial cells. Similar finding was reported by Yam et al. (2009) where TEMF failed to reduce TNF-α production in RAW 264.7 macrophages cells. It can be suggested that TEMF selectively inhibit IL-6 production but not TNF-α.

In this present study, TEMF significantly inhibit protein and gene expression of adhesion molecules (i.e. ICAM-1, VCAM-1 and e-selectin) in human endothelial cells. Similarly, other investigators have reported the ability of TCTs in reducing ICAM-1, VCAM-1 and e-selectin expression in human endothelial cells (Theriault et al., 2002; Naito et al., 2005). Subsequently, the reduction of adhesion molecules by

TEMF (0.3 – 10 μM) further leads to reduce monocytes binding activity to endothelial cells as demonstrated in this present study. It was suggested that, when the adhesion molecule signal is inhibited, leukocytes may still bind to the endothelium but they are not able to undergo transendothelial migration (Valencia & Mills, 2006). The leukocytes that bind to the endothelium but do not complete transendothelial migration are often detached from the endothelium and float away in the blood flow (Cook-Mills & McCary, 2010). Thus, the endothelial cell adhesion molecules and their intracellular signals are a source for intervention in leukocyte recruitment during inflammation and endothelial activation (Cook-Mills & McCary, 2010). This is a very promising finding since adherence of circulating monocytes to the endothelium is the first step in the formation of fatty streak in atherogenesis (Tan, 2005)

NFκB activation is an important mediator for the cytokines and adhesion molecules expression in atherosclerosis. In this present study, NFκB p50 activation was being suppressed by co-incubation of LPS and TEMF at 0.3 – 10 μM in human endothelial cells. Similarly, TEMF was reported to inhibit NFκB p50 activation in rat macrophages cells (Ng & Ko, 2012). Therefore, results from this study indicate that TEMF could exhibit its anti-inflammatory and anti-endothelial activation by suppressing NFκB activity thus resulting in inhibition of adhesion molecule expression.

This present study reported an increment in eNOS protein expression by TEMF at lower concentrations (0.3 - 1.3 μM). Increment of eNOS expression will further lead to increase nitric oxide (NO) (Zhang et al., 2012). Reports on the effects of TEMF on eNOS expression in endothelial cells are scarce. In macrophage cells, it has been reported that TEMF significantly reduced NO production (Ng & Ko, 2012; Yam at al., 2009; Wu et al., 2008). NO production was found to be reduced by TEMF in microglia cells, the resident immune cells of the central nervous system (Tan et al., 2011). The discrepancies of the result may be due to the different cell culture system (macrophage vs. endothelial cells) and the use of different approaches in the experiment protocols.

This present study demonstrates, for the first time, that TEMF co-incubation with LPS attenuates NFκB activation and at the same time increases eNOS protein expression especially at moderate concentration in human endothelial cells. There was a strong correlation observed between eNOS (leading to increase NO production) and NFκB activation (Porcel et al., 2002). It has been demonstrated that the restoration of the functional NO pathway with antioxidant supplementation attenuated the activation of NFκB (Porcel et al., 2002). NO modulates vascular tone, inhibits platelet function, prevents adhesion of leukocytes and reduce proliferation of the tunica intima (Forstermann, 2010). NO also function as an anti-inflammatory agent and depressing leukocyte adhesion (Kuhlencordt et al., 2004). It is postulated that the ability of NO to inhibit protein and gene expression of inflammation and endothelial activation is at least in part mediated via a reduction in NFκB activity and induces transcription of IκBα, an inhibitor of NFκB thus stabilizing the inhibitory NFκB/IκBα complex in the cytosol (Porcel at al., 2002).

Results from this present study indicate that TEMF (TCTs:α-TOC ratio = 70:30%) leads to reduction in protein and gene expression IL-6, ICAM-1, VCAM-1 and e-selectin by stimulated endothelial cells, mediated via downregulation of NFκB and upregulation of eNOS. As TEMF used in this study is composed of α-, β-, γ- and δ-TCT and α-TOC, further investigation was carried out to determine the most potent Vitamin E isomers responsible for the reduction of inflammation, endothelial activation, monocytes binding activity and eNOS upregulation.

5.2 TCT ISOMERS REDUCES INFLAMMATION ENDOTHELIAL ACTIVATION, MONOCYTES BINDING ACTIVITY, NFκB AND eNOS IN ENDOTHELIAL CELLS

This further investigation was carried out to determine which Vitamin E fractions in TEMF were responsible for the inhibition of IL-6, adhesion molecules, monocytes binding activity, NFκB and at the same time increased the eNOS expression. In this study, HUVECs were incubated with LPS together with either α-, β-, γ-, δ- TCT pure isomers or α-TOC at 0.3 – 10 μM concentration for 16 hours prior to analysis for above mention biomarkers. The effects of each pure TCT isomers and α-TOC on protein and IL-6, TNF-α, ICAM-1, VCAM-1, e-selectin, monocytes binding activity, NFκB and eNOS was then evaluated. With those results, the most potent Vitamin E isomers were further determined by performing area under the curve analysis combining all concentrations (0.3 µM – 10 µM).

It has been found that, co-incubation of LPS and all pure TCT isomers (α-, β-, γ- and δ-TCT) at 0.3-10 µM concentrations showed reduction in IL-6, ICAM-1, monocytes binding activity and NFκB activation in human endothelial cells but not for α-TOC. Only γ-TCT and δ -TCT reduces VCAM-1 and e-selectin. Endothelial nitric oxide synthase (eNOS) expression was induced by γ-TCT and δ –TCT but not by α-TCT, β- TCT and α- TOC. TCT isomers failed to reduce TNF- α expression in human endothelial cells. α-TOC failed to significantly reduce any inflammatory and endothelial activation biomarkers and did not lead to the increment eNOS expression in human endothelial cells. These results suggested that the anti-inflammatory and anti-endothelial activation property of that has been shown by TEMF earlier is mainly contributed by TCT isomers but not α-TOC. In fact, α- TOC is capable in attenuating the anti-atherosclerotic benefits potentially shown by TCTs. These data are consistent with previous studies where it has been shown that TCT isomers but not α-TOC reduces VCAM-1, e-selectin and monocytes binding activity in endothelial cells exposed to either 25-hydroxycholesterol or TNF-α (Naito at al., 2005; Choa at al., 2002). To date, it has been reported that all individual TCT isomers are more potent than α-TOC in the reduction of IL-6 expression and NFκB activation in macrophages/monocytes cells but not yet in human endothelial cells (Qureshi et al., 2011). In this present study, it is observed that γ-TCT and δ-TCT induced eNOS expression at both protein and gene expression levels. However, γ-TCT effectively exhibit stronger increment of eNOS protein and gene expression than δ-TCT. In addition, there was a marked increment of eNOS expression by γ-TCT at higher concentrations (2.5 – 10 µM). Previously, it has been reported that γ-TCT acts as a myocardial conditioning agent by activating the eNOS expression (Ikeda et al., 2003). The other observation from this present study is that γ-TCT significantly reduces IL-6, TNF-α, VCAM-1, e-selectin and NFκB gene expression at lower concentrations (0.3 - 1.3µM). In contrast at higher concentrations (2.5 - 10 µM), γ-TCT significantly induced the IL-6, TNF-α, VCAM-1 and NFκB gene expression. However, β- TCT acts in the opposite direction where it reduces VCAM-1 and NFκB gene expression at higher concentrations (2.5 – 10 µM). Therefore, it is suggested that there was a reversal effects of β- vs. γ-TCT in the reduction of VCAM-1 and NFκB gene expression. Each TCT isomers have different effects in terms of suppression in NFκB gene expression. In this present study, it has been observed that α- and γ- TCT reduces NFκB gene expression at low concentrations (0.3 - 1.3 μM) and not at higher concentrations (2.5 – 10 μM). In contrast, β- TCT at higher concentrations (2.5 – 10 μM) reduces NFκB gene expression. δ- TCT reduces NFκB gene expression across all concentrations (0.3 – 10 μM) indicating that δ-TCT is the most effective TCT isomers in the reduction of NFκB gene expression. α- TCT does the opposite direction where it actually increases NFκB gene expression. This present study showed pure TCT isomers are more potent than α-TOC in terms of reducing IL-6, ICAM-1, VCAM-1, e-selectin, monocytes binding activity and inducing eNOS expression in stimulated endothelial cells.

The next observation in this study is to determine the more potent TCT isomers in the reduction of IL-6, ICAM-1, VCAM-1, e-selectin, monocytes binding activity and NFκB and at the same time increases eNOS expression in human endothelial cells. Area under the curve (AUC) analysis reveals that δ-TCT is the most potent vitamin E isomers in reducing protein and gene expression IL-6 with 25.6 % and 73.2 % inhibition respectively which were 3 - 4 folds that of α-TOC. Similarly, δ-TCT has been shown to be the most potent TCT isomers in the reduction of IL-6 expression in different cell culture system (macrophages) (Yam et al., 2009). The researchers found that co-incubation of LPS and TCT isomers for 24 hours reduced IL-6 protein expression and among all TCT isomers, δ-TCT showed the best inhibitory effects.

This present study shows that δ-TCT is the most potent TCT isomers in suppressing protein and gene expression of ICAM-1 with 38.8 % and 76.3 % inhibition which were 1-3 folds that of α-TOC. VCAM-1 protein and gene expression was being reduced effectively by δ-TCT compared to the other TCT isomers with 59.3 % and 88.7 % inhibition respectively. δ-TCT reduces VCAM-1 by 1 – 2 folds better than α-TOC. This present study also shows that, δ-TCT is the most potent TCT isomers for the reduction of e-selectin gene expression (60.8 % inhibition) which was 2 folds that of α-TOC. Besides that, δ-TCT exerted the most profound inhibitory effects on monocytes binding activity compared to the other TCT isomers with 35.7 % inhibition which was 2 folds that of α-TOC. Consistently, Naito et al. (2005)

reported similar finding where δ-TCT act as the most potent TCT isomers for the reduction of VCAM-1 and monocytes binding activity in human endothelial cells exposed to 25-hydroxycholesterol. Choa et al. (2002) reported similar finding where they also found that δ-TCT is the most effective agent for the reduction of VCAM-1, e-selectin and monocytes binding activity in TNF-α stimulated endothelial cells. In that paper, the inhibitory action was reversed by co-incubation with fernosol and geranylgeraniol, suggesting a role for prenylated proteins in the regulation of adhesion molecule and monocytes adhesion. Therefore protein prenylation has been suggested as a possible target point (Theriault et al., 2002). There was an involvement of protein prenylation, via the mevalonate pathway, as a mediator of cytokine-induced expression of adhesion molecule and monocytic cell adherence shown in the previous study (Sadeghi et al., 2000). This possible anti-endothelial activation mechanism of action has been derived from the previous studies that reported the ability of HMG CoA reductase inhibitors to interfere the protein prenylation and lowering the production of adhesion molecules (Weber et al., 1997). Protein prenylation is a post-transcriptional event that regulates the activity of small G proteins such as Ras and Rho by modifying its structure with farnesyl or geranylgeranyl groups (Sinensky & Lutz, 1992). Figure 5.1 shows the possible anti-endothelial activation mechanisms of tocotrienols via the inhibition of HMG CoA reductase and protein prenylation pathway.

Previously, it has also been shown that the reduction of adhesion molecule expression and monocytes binding activity are NFκB dependent (Theriault et al., 2002). Subsequently, this present study has demonstrated that NFκB p50 binding activity and gene expression was effectively suppressed by δ-TCT with 22.4 % and 53.6 % inhibition respectively which was 2-3 folds of that α-TOC. Previously, α-TCT was reported to effectively reduce NFκB activation in TNF-α stimulated endothelial cells (Theriault et al., 2002). It has been suggested that TCT blocks the NFκB activation through the ability of TCT in inhibiting the phosphorylation of IκB by IKK complex leading to decrease of IκB complex degradation (Nasaretnam & Meganathan, 2011). When the IκB complex degradation is decreased, the translocation of NFκB into the nucleus is also being suppressed leading to further reduction of NFκB activation (Ng & Ko, 2012).

γ-TCT is the most potent TCT isomers in increasing eNOS protein and gene expression with 37.5 % and 757.7 % increment which was 1 - 17 folds of that α-TOC. A similar finding was reported by Das et al. (2005) where among all TCT isomers, γ-TCT is the most potent TCT isomers in inducing the eNOS expression. Ikeda et al. (2003) reported that γ-TCT acts as myocardial conditioning agent by activating the eNOS expression. As a consequence, eNOS enhances NO production, leading to vasodilatation and cardioprotection from ischemic phase (Ikeda et al., 2003). In this present study, it has been observed that at higher concentrations (2.5 – 10 μM), γ-TCT induces eNOS and NFκB gene expression. At lower concentrations (0.3 – 1.3 μM), γ- TCT effectively reduces NFκB gene expression. Base on this observation, it is suggested that γ- TCT is a potent antioxidant at high concentrations and at low concentrations; it is a potent anti-inflammatory agent. γ- TCT exhibits potent anti-oxidant activity eight fold higher than that as an anti-inflammatory agent. In comparison with the other TCT isomers, this study demonstrated that δ-TCT is the most potent and effective anti-inflammatory and anti-endothelial activation agent. In this study, it has been shown that the effective anti-inflammatory and anti-endothelial activation action of δ- TCT are mediated by NFκB pathway. Other investigator has also demonstrated that the potency of δ-TCT is due to the number of methyl group (one) which abolishes regulatory activity with respect to the HMG-CoA reductase degradation and sterol regulatory element-binding proteins (SREBP-2) processing (Qureshi et al., 2011). Naito et al. (2005) has demonstrated that the highest intracellular concentration of Vitamin E analogues in endothelial cells is δ- TCT compared to α- TCT and γ- TCT. These suggest that the superior anti-endothelial activation property of TCT isomers is possibly due to their intracellular concentrations (Noguchi et al, 2003).

This present study indicates that TEMF and TCT isomers are a more potent and effective anti-inflammatory and anti-endothelial activation agent than α-TOC. α-TOC does not play any role in inhibiting the inflammation and endothelial activation in LPS-stimulated human endothelial cells. In fact, α-TOC does the opposite direction where it enhances IL-6, ICAM-1, e-selectin expression, NFκB activation and monocyte binding activity. In addition, α-TOC does not have any beneficial effects in the suppression of VCAM-1 expression and eNOS induction. In this study, pure TCT particularly γ- and δ- isomers clearly exhibited to have greater potency than TEMF (TCTs:α-TOC ratio = 70:30 %) by showing greater reduction of IL6, ICAM-1, VCAM-1, NFκB and monocyte binding activity (MBA). In addition, γ- and δ TCT isomers have greater potency than TEMF in inducing eNOS expression in LPS stimulated HUVECs. This enhances observation that pure TCT isomers have beneficial effects in terms of inflammation and endothelial activation and α- TOC have detrimental effects to TCT benefits. TCTs in combination with α-TOC still have the goodies but inferior to that pure TCT particularly γ- and δ- isomers. α-TOC has been shown to interfere with the functions and benefits of TCTs for example in lipid lowering activity (Qureshi et al., 1996). Studies are compared with regards to varying amounts of α-TOC content in TCT mixtures, and are found to yield better results if α-TOC is low or absent (Qureshi et al., 1996; Qureshi et al., 2011). It has been suggested that for cardiovascular disease, the rule-of-thumb for an effective composition is greater than 60 % of γ- and δ TCT isomers and 0 - 15 % α-TOC (Qureshi et al., 1996).

The presence of isoprenoid side chain in TCT is accounted for the superior activity of TCT over TOC. Structurally, TCTs and TOCs can be distinguished by their side chains, and it has been reported that the unsaturated side chain of TCT allows it to pass through cell membranes more efficiently and at a faster rate than the saturated phytyl side chain of TOCs. For this reason, the greater anti-inflammatory, anti endothelial activation may be due in part to their effective incorporation into endothelial cells (Miyazawa et al., 2008).

FIGURE 5.1

The Possible Anti-Endothelial Activation of TCTs via the Inhibition of 3-hydroxy-3-Methylglutaryl Coenzyme A (HMG CoA) Reductase and Protein Prenylation Pathway. The Prenylated Side-Chain of TCTs Induces Prenyl Pyrophosphate Pyrophosphatase Which Catalyses the Dephosphorylation of Farnesyl, Resulting in an Increase in Cellular Farnesol. Farnesol Down-Regulates HMG-CoA Reductase Activity Post-Transcriptionally by Increasing Enzyme Degradation, Without Reducing HMG-CoA gene expression. The Reduction of Farnesyl Pyrophosphate (PP) and Geranylgeraniol PP Interfere Protein Prenylation Pathway Leading to Suppression of NFκB Activation and Adhesion Molecule Production. Adapted from Theriault et al. (1999) and Frank et al. (2012).

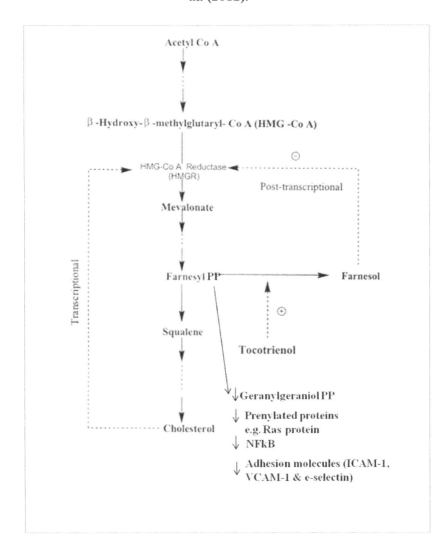

CHAPTER SIX
CONCLUSION

This study adds knowledge to the scarcity of published studies on TCTs and their anti-inflammatory effects in relation to atherosclerosis. To date, studies on the anti-inflammatory TCTs were more focused on the cancer chemoprevention and treatment but very few have reported on TCTs as an anti-atherosclerotic agent. Tocotrienols (TCTs) exhibits its anti-atherosclerotic property through NFκB reduce activation leading to decreased IL-6 expression and subsequently suppressed ICAM-1, VCAM-1 and e-selectin expression. Then, it leads to the suppression of monocyte adherence to endothelial cells. Furthermore, this present study clearly showed the ability of TCTs in attenuating NFκB activation and increases eNOS expression in human endothelial cells. This will provide better cardioprotective effects. Pure TCT isomers especially delta isomer (δ- TCT) have an effective anti-inflammatory and anti-endothelial activation properties which is mediated via NFκB reduce activation. In addition, γ-TCT is the most potent TCT isomers in inducing eNOS expression. Tocotrienol inhibitory effects on monocytes-endothelial adhesion, a key event in atherogenesis will further render anti-atherosclerotic and cardioprotective benefits of TCT. In contrast, this present study clearly reveals that pure α-TOC does not lead to reduction in inflammation and endothelial activation. In fact, pure α-TOC appears to be detrimental as an anti-atherosclerotic agent where it upregulates IL-6, ICAM-1 and NFκB, and downregulates eNOS gene expression in addition enhancing monocyte adherence to endothelial cells. These anti-atherosclerotic mechanisms of pure α-TOC may in part explain the lack of benefits and detrimental effects of α-TOC in clinical trials involving CAD subjects (Gee, 2011). These interesting findings may also explain the reduced beneficial effects of TEMF compared to pure TCTs where their benefits may be inhibited by the presence of α-TOC. Therefore, it is hence timely for pure TCT isomers and TEMF to be evaluated clinically to fully explore their therapeutic potential in view of numerous *in vitro* and *in vivo* studies, and to a very limited extend human intervention clinical trials. Therefore, given the important roles of inflammation and endothelial activation in the pathogenesis of atherosclerosis, and by virtue of the potent anti-inflammatory and anti-endothelial activation effects of TCTs and TEMF, there is a strong potential of TCTs in the prevention of atherosclerosis and thus as an anti-atherosclerotic agent. TCT may have therapeutic potential in atherosclerosis-related diseases such as coronary artery disease (CAD), peripheral vascular disease (PVD), stroke and metabolic syndrome and in environment with enhanced inflammation such as spaceflight travel.

REFERENCES

Altman, R. (2004). Risk factor in coronary atherosclerosis athero-inflammation: the meeting point. *Thrombosis Journal, 1,* 4-8.

Alwan A, T. A., Cowan, M., & Riley, L. (2011). *Global status report on noncommunicable diseases.*

Amar, J., Fauvel., J., Drouet, L., Ruidavets, J.B., & Perret, B. (2006). Interleukin 6 is associated with subclinical atherosclerosis: a link with soluble intercellular adhesion molecule-1. *Journal of Hypertension, 24,* 1083-1088.

Amplavanar, N. T, Gurpreet, K., Salmiah, M. S., & Odhayakumar, N. (2010). Prevalence of cardiovascular disease risk factors among attendees of the Batu 9, Cheras Health Centre, Selangor, Malaysia. *Malaysian Medical Journal, 65*(3), 166-172.

Anderson, R. K., Hushen, J., Cameron, D. F., & Tran-Son-Tay, R. (2003). Effects of simulated microgravity culture technology on cell-cell and cell-substrate adhesion. *Summer Bioengineering Conference*, June 25-29, Sonesta Beach Resort in Key Biscayne, Florida.

Azman, W., & Sim, K. H. (2006). Annual Report of the National Cardiovascular Disease-Acute Coronary Syndrome: National Registry Malaysia Kuala Lumpur.

Babu, N. P., Pandikumar, P., & Ignacimuthu, S. (2009). Anti-inflammatory activity of Albizia lebbeck Benth., an ethnomedicinal plant, in acute and chronic animal models of inflammation. *Journal of Ethnopharmacology, 125* (2), 356-360.

Bach, F. H., Robson, S. C, Ferran, C, Winkler, H., Millan, M., Stuhlmeier, K. M., Vanhove, B., Blakely, M. L., van der Werf W. J., & Hofer, E. (1994). Endothelial cell activation and thromboregulation during xenograft rejection. *Immunological Reviews*, *141,* 5-30.

Baliarsingh, S., Beg, Z. H., & Ahmad, J. (2005). The therapeutic impacts of tocotrienols in type 2 diabetic patients with hyperlipidaemia. *Atherosclerosis, 182* (2), 367-374.

Baqai, F. P., Gridley, D. S., Slater, J. M., Luo-Owen, X., Stodieck, L. S., Ferguson, V., Chapes, S. K., & Pecaut, M. J. (2009). Effects of spaceflight on innate immune function and antioxidant gene expression. *Journal of Applied Physiology 106*(6), 1935-42.

Beinke, S. O. & Ley, S. C. (2004). Functions of NF-κB1 and NF-κB2 in immune cell biology. *Biochemical Journal, 382,* 393-409.

Bermudez, E. A., Rifai, N., Buring, J. E., Manson, J. E., & Ridker, P. M. (2002). Relation between markers of systemic vascular inflammation and smoking in women. *American Journal of Cardiology,* 89, 1117-1119.

Bevilacqua, M. F., Stengelin, S., Gimbrone, M. A., & Seed, B. (1989). Endothelial leukocyte adhesion molecule-1: an inducible receptor to neutrophils related to complement regulatory proteins and lectins. *Science, 243,* 1160-1165.

Bienke, S., & Ley, S. C. (2004). Functions of NF-κB1 and NF-κB2 in immune cell biology. *Biochemical Journal, 382,* 393–409.

Black, T. M., Wang, P., Maeda, N., & Coleman, R. A. (2000). Palm tocotrienols protect ApoE +/- mice from diet induced atheroma formation. *Journal of Nutrition,* 130, 2420-2426.

Blake G. J., & Ridker P. M. (2002). Inflammatory bio-markers and cardiovascular risk prediction. *Journal of Internal Medicine, 252*(4), 283-294.

Blake G. J., & Ridker P. M. (2002). Tumour necrosis factor-α an inflammatory biomarkers and atherogenesis. *European Heart Journal, 23,* 345-347.

Blann, A. D., Admiral, J., & McCollum, C. N. (1996). Circulating Endothelial Cell/Leukocyte Adhesion Molecules in Ischaemic Heart Disease. *British Journal of Haematology, 95,* 263-265.

Bouis, D, Hospers, G.A., Meijer, C., Molema, G., & Mulder, N.H. (2001). Endothelium *in vitro*: a review of human vascular endothelial cell lines for blood vessel-related research. *Angiogenesis, 4*(2), 91-102.

Branen, L., Lars, H., Nitulescu, M., Bengtsson, E., Nilsson, J., & Jovinge S. (2004). Inhibition of tumor necrosis factor-α reduces atherosclerosis in Apolipoprotein E knockout mice. *Arteriosclerosis, Thrombosis and Vascular Biology, 24,* 2137-2142.

Brigelius-Flohe, R. (2007). Adverse effects of vitamin E by induction of drug metabolism. Genes Nutrition, 2, 249-256.

Buravkova L., Romanov Y., Rykova M., Grigorieva, O., & Merzlikina, N. (2005). Cell-to-cell interactions in changed gravity: Ground-based and flight experiments. *Acta Astronautica,* 67-74.

Buravkova, L. B., & Romanov, Y. A. (2001). The role of cytoskeleton in cell changes under condition of simulated microgravity. *Acta Astronautica, 48*(5-12), 647-650.

Bustin, S. A., Benes, V., Garson, J. A., Hellemans, J., Huggett, J., Kubista, M., Mueller, R., Nolan, T., Pfaffl, M. W., Shipley, G. L., Vandesompele, J., & Wittwer, C. T. (2009). The MIQE Guidelines: Minimum Information for Publication of Quantitative Real-Time PCR Experiments. *Clinical Chemistry, 55*(4), 611-622.

Carlsson, S. I. M., Bertilaccio M. T. S., Ballabio E., & Maier, J. A. M. (2003). Endothelial stress by gravitational unloading: effects on cell growth and cytoskeletal organization. *Biochimica et Biophysica Acta, 1642,* 173-179.

Champagne, B., Tremblay, P., Cantin, A., & St Pierre, Y. (1998). Proteolytic cleavage of ICAM-1 by human neutrophil elastase. *The Journal of Immunology, 161,* 6398-6405.

Chao, J. T., Gapor, A., & Theriault, A. (2002) Inhibitory effect of delta-tocotrienol, a HMG-CoA reductase inhibitor, mononocyte endothelial cell adhesion. *Journal of Nutritional Science & Vitaminology, 48,* 332-337.

Chatterjee, A., & Catravas, J. D. (2008). Endothelial nitric oxide (NO) and its pathophysiologic regulation. *Vascular Pharmacology., 49* (4-6), 134–140.

Chen C, et al. (1999). High affinity very late antigen -4 subsets expressed on T-cells are mandatory for spontaneous adhesion strengthening but not for rolling VCAM-1 in shear flow. *The Journal of Immunology, 162,* 1084-1095.

Chen, S. C., Chang, Y. L., Wang, D. L., & Cheng, J. J. (2006). Herbal remedy magnolol suppress IL-6 induced STAT-3 activation and gene expression in endothelial cells. British *Journal of Pharmacology, 148,* 226-232.

Chen, Z. J. (2005). Ubiquitin signalling in the NF-kappaB pathway. *Nature Cell Biology, 7*(8), 758-765.

Chia, S., Qadan, M., Newton, R., Ludlam, C. A., Fox, K. A. A., & Newby, D. E. (2003). Intra-Arterial Tumor Necrosis Factor-a Impairs Endothelium-Dependent Vasodilatation c and Stimulates Local Tissue Plasminogen Activator Release in Humans. *Arteriosclerosis, Thrombosis, and Vascular Biology 23*, 695-701.

Cines, D. B., Pollak, E.S., Buck, C.A, Loscalzo, J., Zimmerman, G. A., & McEver, R. P. (1998). Endothelial cells in the pathophysiology of vascular disorders. *Blood*, 3527-3561.

Clement, G. (2005). The maintenance of physiological function in humans during spaceflight, *International Sport Med Journal*, *6*(4), 185-198.

Coccia, E. M., Russo, N. D., Stellaci, E., Testa, U., Marziali, G., & Battistini, A. (1999). STAT-1 activation during monocyte to macrophage maturation: role of adhesion molecule. *International Immunology, 11,* 1075-1083.

Cockerill, G. W., Rye, K. A., Gamble, J. R., Vadas, M. A., & Barter, P. J. (1995). High-density lipoproteins inhibit cytokine-induced expression of endothelial cell adhesion molecules. *Arteriosclerosis, Thrombosis & Vascular Biology, 15,* 1987-1994.

Constans, J., & Conri, C. (2006). Circulating markers of endothelial function in cardiovascular disease. *Clinica Chimica Acta, 368,* 33-47.

Cook-Mills, J. M., & McCary, C. A. (2010). Isoforms of vitamin E differentially regulate inflammation. *Endocr Metab Immune Disord Drug Targets, 10* (4), 348-366.

Cotran, R. S. (1989). Endothelial Cells. In *Kelly's Textbook of Rheumatology* (Ruddy S, Harris ED Jr, Sledge CB, eds. Vol 1, 389-415, W.B Saunders, Company Philadelphia.

Cotrupi, S., Ranzani, D., & Maier, J. A. A. (2005). Impact of modeled microgravity on microvascular endothelial cells. *Biochimica et Biophysica Acta, 1746,* 163-168.

Croute F, Gaubin Y., Pianezzi B., Soleihavoup J.P. (1995). Effects of hypergravity on the cell shape and on the organization of cytoskleteon and extracellular matrix molecules on *in vitro* human dermal fibroblasts. *Microgravity Science and Technology, 8,* 118.

Cybulski, M. I., & Gimbrone M. A. (1991). Endothelial expression of a mononuclear leukocyte adhesion molecule during atherogenesis. *Science. 251,* 788–791.

Das, S., Powell, S. R., Wang, P., Divald, A., Nesaretnam, K., Tosaki, A., Cordis, G. A., et al. (2005). Cardioprotection with palm tocotrienol: antioxidant activity of tocotrienol is linked with its ability to stabilize proteasomes. *American Journal of Physiology - Heart and Circulatory Physiology, 289,* 361-367.

Daxecker, H., Raab, M., Markovic, S., Karimi, A., Griesmacher, A., & Mueller, M. M. (2002). Endothelial Adhesion Molecule Expression in an *in vitro* model of inflammation. *Clinica Chimica Acta, 325,* 171-175.

De Meyer, G. R., & Herman, A. G. (1997). Vascular endothelial dysfunction. *Progress in Cardiovascular Diseases, 39,* 325-42.

Dieriks, B., Vos, W. D., Messen, G., Oostveld, K. V., Meyer, T. D., Ghardi, M., et al. (2009). High content analysis of Human Fibroblast cell cultures after exposure to space radiation. *Radiation Research, 172*(4), 423-436.

Ding, B. S., Dziublam, T., Shuvaev, V. V., Muro, S., Muzykantov, V. R. (2006). Advance drug delivery systems that target the vascular endothelium. *Molecular Interventions, 6,* 98-112.

Dong, Z. M., Chapman, S. M., Brown, A. A., Frenette, P. S., Hynes, R. O., & Wagner D. (1998). The combined role of p-selectin and e-selectin in Atherosclerosis. *Journal of Clinical Investigations, 102,* 145-152.

D'Orleans, J. P., Mitchell, J. A., Wood, E. G., Hecker, M., & Vane, J. R. (1992). Comparison of the release of vasoactive factors from venous and arterial bovine cultured endothelial cells. Canadian Journal of Physiology & Pharmacology, 70(5), 687-694.

Dutta, A., & Dutta, S. (2003). Vitamin E and its Role in the Prevention of Atherosclerosis and Carcinogenesis: A Review. *Journal of the American College of Nutrition, 22*(4), 258-268.

Ebong, P. E., Owu, D. U., & Isong, E. U. (1999). Influence of palm oil (*Elaesis guineensis*) on health. *Plant Foods for Human Nutrition (Formerly Qualitas Plantarum), 53*(3), 209-222.

Enginar, H., Cemek, M., Karaca, T., & Unak, P. (2007). Effect of grape seed extract on lipid peroxidation, antioxidant activity and peripheral blood lymphocytes in rats exposed to x-radiation. *Phytotherapy Research, 21*(11), 1029-35.

Eppihimer, M. J., Wolitzky, B., Anderson, D. C., Labow, M. A., & Granger, D. N. (1996). Heterogeneity of expression of E and P-selectin *in vivo*. *Circulation Research, 79,* 560-569.

Fan, J. & Watanabe, T. (2003). Inflammatory reactions in the pathogenesis of atherosclerosis. *Journal of Atherosclerosis and Thrombosis, 10,* 63-71.

Feairheller, D. L., Park, J. Y., Rizzo, V., Kim, B., & Brown, M. D. (2011). Racial differences in the responses to shear stress in human umbilical vein endothelial cells. *Clinical and Translational Science, 4,* 32-37.

Fergusona, L. R. (2010). Chronic inflammation and mutagenesis. *Mutation Research 690,* 3-11.

Fish, J. E., Matouk, C. C., Rachlis, A., Lin, S., Tai, S. C., D'Abreo, C., Marsden, P. A. (2005). The expression of endothelial nitrix-oxide synthase is control by a-cell specific histone code. The *Journal of Biological Chemistry, 280*(26), 24824-24838.

Fong K. (2004). The next small step. *Biomedical Journal, 329,* 1441-1444.

Forstermann, U. (2010). Nitric oxide and oxidative stress in vascular disease. *Pfluegers Archiv, 459,* 923-939.

Francisco, G., Hernandez, C., & Simo, R. (2006). Serum markers of vascular inflammation in dyslipidemia. *Clinica Chimica Acta, 369,* 1-16.

Frank, J., Chin, X. W. D., Schrader, C., Eckert, G. P., & Rimbach, G. (2012). Do tocotrienols have potential as neuroprotective dietary factors? *Ageing Research Reviews, 11,* 163- 180.

Fries, J. W., Williams, A. J., Atkins, R. C., Newman, W., Lipscomb, M. F., & Collins, T. (1993). Expression of VCAM-1 and E-selectin in an *in vivo* model of endothelial activation. *American Journal of Pathology, 143,* 725-37.

Fruchart, J. C., Nierman, M. C., Stroes, E. S. G., Kastelein J. J. P., & Duriez, P. (2003). Atherosclerosis: Evolving Vascular Biology and Clinical Implications. *Circulation, 109* (III), **15- 19**

Galkina, E., & Ley, K. (2007). Leukocyte influx in atherosclerosis. *Current Drug Targets, 8*(12), 1239-1248.

Gaziano, T. A., Bitton, A., Anand, S., Gessel, S. A., & Murphy, A. (2010). Growing Epidemic of Coronary Heart Disease in Low- and Middle- Income Countries. *Current Problems in Cardiology, 35*(2), 72-115.

Gee, P. T. (2011). Unleashing the untold and misunderstood observations on vitamin E. *Genes Nutrition, 6* (1), 5-16.

Gersh, B. J., Sliwa, K., Mayosi, B. M., & Yusuf, S. (2010). The epidemic of cardiovascular disease in the developing world: global implications. *European Heart Journal, 31*, 642–648

Glass, C. K., & Witztum, J. L. (2001) Atherosclerosis. The road ahead. *Cell, 104,* 503-516.

Goodwin, B. L., Pendleton, L. C., Levy, M. M., Solomonson, L. P. & Eichler, D. C. (2007). Tumor necrosis factor-α reduces argininosuccinate synthase expression and nitric oxide production in aortic endothelial cells. *American Journal of Physiology - Heart and Circulatory Physiology, 293*, H1115–H1121.

Griffoni, C., Molfetta, S. D., Fantozzi, L., Zanetti, C., Pippia, P., Tomasi, V., & Spisni, E. (2011). Modifications of proteins secreted by endothelial cells during model low gravity exposure. *Journal of Cellular Biochemistry, 112,* 265-272.

Grosse, J., Wehland, M., Pietsch, J., Ma, X., Ulbrich, C., Schulz, H., Saar, K., Hübner, N., Hauslage, J., Hemmersbach, R., Braun, M., van Loon, J., Vagt, N., Infanger, M, Eilles, C., Egli, M., Richter, P., Baltz, T., Einspanier, R., Sharbati, S., & Grimm D. (2012). Short-term weightlessness produced by parabolic flight maneuvers altered gene expression patterns in human endothelial cells. *FASEB Journal, 26* (2), 639-655.

Grove D. S., Pishak, S. A., & Mastro A. M. (1995). The effect of a 10-day space flight on the function, phenotype, and adhesion molecule expression of splenocytes and lymph node lymphocytes. *Experimental of Cellular Research, 219* (1), 102-109.

Guilder, V. G. P., Hoetzer, G. L., Greiner, J. J., Stauffer, B. L., & Desouza, C. A. (2006). Influence of metabolic syndrome on biomarkers of oxidative stress and inflammation in obese adults. *Obesity, 14* (12), 2127-2131.

Guray, U., Erbay, A. R., Guray, Y., Yilmaz, M. B., Boyaci, A. A, Sasmaz, H., Korkmaz, S., & Kütük, E. (2004). Levels of soluble adhesion molecules in various clinical presentation of coronary atherosclerosis. *International Journal of Cardiology, 96*, 235-240.

Hansson, G. K. (2001). Immune mechanism in atherosclerosis. *Arteriosclerosis Thrombosis & Vascular Biology, 21,* 1876-1890.

Hansson, G. K., & Hermansson, A. (2011). The immune system in atherosclerosis. *Nature Immunology, 12*, 204-212.

Harris, T. B., Ferrucci, L., Tracy, R. P., Corti, M. C., Wacholder, S., Ettinger, W. H. Jr., et al., (1999). Associations of elevated interleukin-6 and C-reactive proteins with mortality in the elderly. *American Journal of Medicine, 106*, 506-512.

Harrison, D.G. (1997). Cellular and molecular mechanisms of endothelial cell dysfunction. *Journal of Clinical Investigations, 100,* 2153.

Hedner, T., Hansson, L., & Himmelmann, A. (2000). Endothelial dysfunction – a challenge for hypertension research. *Blood Press,* 2-3.

Hegewisch, S., Weh, H. J., & Hossfeld, D. K. (1990). TNF- α induced cardiomyopathy. *Lancet, 335*(8684), 294-305.

Heinrich, P. C., Behrmann, I., Haan, S., Hermanns, H. M., Muller-Newen, G., & Schaper, F. (2003). Principles of interleukin (IL)-6-type cytokine signaling and its regulation. *Journal of Biochemistry, 374*, 1-20.

Hickey, M. J. (2001). Role of inducible nitric oxide synthase in the regulation of leukocyte recruitment. *Clinical Science, 100,* 1-12.

Hillis, G.S. (2003). Soluble integrin adhesion receptors and atherosclerosis: much heat and a little light. *Journal of Human Hypertension, 17,* 449-453.

Hood, R. L., Ong, A. S. H., Niki, E., Packer, L. (Eds.). (1996). *Tocotrienols and cholesterol metabolism. In:. Nutrition, lipids, health, and diseases.* Champaign, IL: AOCS Press.

Huang, P. L. & Lo, E. H. (1998). Genetic analysis of NOS isoforms using nNOS and eNOS knockout animals. *Progress in Brain Research, 118,* 13.

Hughes-Fulford M. (2011). To infinity and beyond! Human spaceflight and life science. *The FASEB Journal, 25,* 2858-2864.

Hunt, B. J., & Jurd, K. M. (1998). Endothelial cell activation. A central pathophysiological process. *Biomedical Journal, 316,* 1328-1329.

Ikeda, S., Tohyama, T., Yoshimura, H., Hamamura, K., Abe, K., & Yamashita K. (2003). Dietary alpha-tocopherol decreases alpha-tocotrienol but not gamma-tocotrienol concentration in rats. *Journal of Nutrition, 133,*428-434.

Ikeda, U., Ikeda, M., Ikeda, Y., Seino, M., Takahashi, S., & Shimada, K. (1992). Interleukin-6 gene transcripts are expressed in atherosclerotics lesions of genetically hyperlipidemic rabbits. *Atherosclerosis, 92,* 213-218.

Infanger, M., Ulbrich, C., Baatout, S., Wehland, M., Kreutz, R., Bauer, J., Grosse, J., Vadrucci, S., Cogoli, A., Derradji, H., Neefs, M., Küsters, S., Spain, M., Paul, M., & Grimm, D. (2007). Modeled gravitational unloading induced downregulation of endothelin-1 in human endothelial cells. *Journal of Cellular Biochemistry, 15,* 101(6), 1439-55.

Ingber, D. (1999). How cells (might) sense microgravity. *FASEB Journal, 13,* S3-S15.

Ito, H., Oshima, A., Inoue, M., Ohto, N., Nakasuga, K., Kaji, Y., Maruyama, T., & Nishioka, K. (2002). Weight Reduction Decreases Soluble Cellular Adhesion Molecules in Obese Women, *Clinical Experimental Pharmacology & Physiology, 29,* 399-404.

Jaffe, E. A., Nachman, R.L., Becker C. G., & Miinick, R. (1973). Culture of human endothelial cells derived from umbilical veins identification by morphologic and immunologic criteria. *The Journal of Clinical Investigation, 52,* 2745-2756.

Jefferson, A., Ruparelia, N., & Choudhury, R. P. (2013). Exogenous Microparticles of Iron Oxide Bind to Activated Endothelial Cells but, Unlike Monocytes, Do Not Trigger an Endothelial Response. *Theranostics, 3*(6), 428-436.

Jasperse J. L., Woodman, C. R., Price, E.M., Hasser, E. M., & Laughlin, M. H. (1999). Hindlimb unweighting decreases eNOS gene expression and eNOS endothelium dependent dilatation in rat soleus feed arteries. *Journal of Applied Physiology, 87*(4), 1476-82.

Jung, C. K., Chung, S., Lee, Y. Y., Hwang S. H., Kang C. S., & Lee, K. Y. (2005). Monocyte adhesion to endothelial cells increases with hind-limb unloading in rats. *Aviation, Space & Environmental Medicine, 76* (8), 720-5.

Kaileh, M., & Sen, R. (2011).Role of NF-kappa B in the anti-inflammatory effects of tocotrienols. *Journal of the American College of Nutrition, 29* (3 suppl), 334S -339S.

Kacena, M. A., Todd, P., & Landis, W .J. (2003). Osteoblasts subjected to spaceflight and simulated space shuttle launch conditions. *In Vitro Cellular & Developmental Biology, Animal, 39*(10), 454-9.

Kamal, E. A., & Appelqvist, L. (1996). The chemistry and antioxidant properties of tocopherols and tocotrienols. *Lipids,* 31, 671-701.

Kamat, J. P., Sarma, H. D., Devasagayam, T. P. A, Nasaretnam, K., & Basiron, Y. (1997). Tocotrienols from palm oil as effective inhibitors of protein oxidation and lipid peroxidation in rat liver microsomes. *Molecular and Cellular Biochemistry, 170,* 131-138.

Kansas, G. S. (1996). Selectines and their ligans: current concepts and controversies. *Blood, 88,* 3259-3287.

Kanters, E., Gjibels, M. J. J., Made, I. V. D., Vergouwe, M.N., Heeringa, P., et al. (2004). Hematopoietic NFκB1 deficiency results in small atherosclerotic lesions with an inflammatory phenotype. *Blood, 103,* 934-940.

Kapitonova, M. Y., Nawawi, H., Froemming, G. R. A., Kuznetsov, S. L., Muid, S., & Manaf, A. (2012). Image-analysis of the structural changes in the endothelial cells during space flight, *Morfologiia, 141* (N3) 70-71.

Kawashima, S., & Yokoyama, M. (2004). Dysfunction of endothelial nitric oxide synthase and atherosclerosis. *Arteriosclerosis Thrombosis & Vascular Biology, 24,* 998.

Khanna, S., Patel, V., Rink, C., Roy, S., & Sen, C. K. (2005). Delivery of orally supplemented alpha-tocotrienol to vital organs of rats and tocopherol-transport protein deficient mice. *Free Radical Biology & Medicine, 39,* 1310-1319.

Khosla, P., Patel, V., Whinter, J. M., Khanna, S., Rakhkovskaya, M., Roy, S., Sen, C. K. (2006). Postprandial levels of the natural vitamin E tocotrienol in human circulation. *Antioxidants and Redox Signalling,* 8(5-6), 1059-1068.

Klingenberg, R., & Hansson, G. K. (2009). Treating inflammation in atherosclerotic cardiovascular disease:emerging therapies. *European Heart Journal, 30,* 2838-2844.

Koenig, W., & Khuseyinova, N. (2007). Biomarkers of Atherosclerotic Plaque Instability and Rupture. *Arteriosclerosis Thrombosis & Vascular Biology, 27,* 15-26.

Kuhlencordt, P. J., Rosel, E., Gerszten, R. E., Ruiz, M. M., Dombkowski, D., Atkinson, W. J., et al. (2004). Role of endothelial nitric oxide synthase in endothelial activation: insights from eNOS knockout endothelial cells. *American Journal of Physiology - Cell Physiology, 286,* C1195-C1202.

Kume, N., Cybulsky, M. I., & Gimbrone, M. A. (1992). Lysosphosphatidylcholine, a component of atherogenic lipoproteins, induces mononuclear leukocyte adhesion molecules in cultured human and rabbit arterial endothelial cells. *Journal of Clinical Investigation, 90,* 1138-1144.

Kumei, Y., Shimokawa, H., Katano, H., Hara, E., Akiyama, H., Hirano, M., Mukai, C., Nagaoka, S., Whitson, P. A., & Sams, C. F. (1996). Microgravity induces prostaglandin E_2 and interleukin-6 production in normal rat osteoblasts: role in bone demineralization. *Journal of Biotechnology, 47 (2-3),* 313-24.

Kunkel, E. J., & Ley, K. (1996). Distinct phenotype of e-selectin deficient mice, e-Selectin is required for slow leukocyte rolling *In Vivo*. *Circulation Research, 79,* 1196-1204.

Kvietys, P. R., & Granger, D. N. (1997). Endothelial cell monolayers as a tool for studying microvascular pathophysiology. *American Journal of Physiology - Gastrointestinal and Liver Physiology, 273,* G1189-G1199.

Kwon, O., Tranter, M., Jones, W. K., Sankovic, J. M., & Banerjee, R. K. (2009). Differential translocation of nuclear factor-kappaB in a cardiac muscle cell line under gravitational changes. *Journal of Biomechanical Engineering, 131*(6), 064503.

Lawson, C., & Wolf S. (2009). ICAM-1 signaling in endothelial cells. *Pharmacological Reports, 61,* 22-32.

Leeuw K. D., Sanders, J. S., Stegeman, C., Smit, A., Kallenberg, C. G., & Bijl, M. (2005). Accelerated atherosclerosis in patients with Wegener's granulomatosis. *Annals of Rheumatology Disease, 64,* 753-759.

Leeuwenberg, J. F., Smeets, E. F., Neefjes, J. J., Shaffer, M. A., Cinek, T., Jeunhomme, T. M., Ahern, T. J., & Buurman, W. A. (1992). E-selectin and intercellular adhesion-molecule-1 are released by activated human endothelial cells *in vitro. Immunology, 77,* 543-549.

Leonarduzzi, G., Gamba, P., Gargiulo, S., Biasi, F., & Poli, G. (2012). Inflammation-related gene expression by lipid oxidation-derived products in the progression of atherosclerosis. *Free Radical Biology & Medicine, 52,* 19-34.

Lewis, D. R., Kamisoglu, K., York, A. W., & Moghe, P. V. (2011). Polymer-based therapeutics: nanoassemblies and nanoparticles for management of atherosclerosis. *WIREs Nanomed Nanobiotechnol, 3,* 400-420.

Ley, K., & Yuqing, Huo. (2001). VCAM-1 is critical in atherosclerosis. *The Journal of Clinical Investigation, 107*(10), 1209-1210.

Li, F., Tan. W., Kang, Z., & Wong, C. W. (2010). Tocotrienol enriched palm oil prevents atherosclerosis through modulating the activities of peroxisome proliferators-activated receptors. *Atherosclerosis, 211,* 278–282

Li, H., Cylbulsky, M. I., Gimbrone, M. A., & Libby, P. (1993). An atherogenic diet rapidly induces VCAM-1, a cytokine-reguatable mononuclear leukocyte adhesion molecule, in rabbit aortic endothelium. *Arteriosclerosis Thrombosis, 13,* 197-204.

Lim, S. S., Gaziano, T. A., Gakidou, E., Reddy, K. S., Farzadfar, F., Lozano, R., & Rodgers, A. (2007). Prevention of cardiovascular disease in high-risk individuals in low-income and middle-income countries: health effects and costs. *Lancet, 370,* 2054–2062.

Lim, Y. C., Snapp, K., Kansas, G. S., Camphausen, R., Ding, H., & Luscinskas, F. W. (1998). Important contributions of p-selectin glycoprotein ligand-1 mediated secondary capture to human monocyte adhesion to p-selectin, e-selectin and TNF- α activated endothelium under flow *in vitro. Journal of Immunology, 161,* 2501-2508.

Liyama, K., Hajra, L., & Liyama, M. (1999). Patterns of vascular cell adhesion molecule -1 and intercellular adhesion molecule -1 in rabbit and mouse atherosclerotic lesions and at sites predisposed to lesion formation. *Circulation Research, 85,* 199-207.

Lishnevskii, A. E. , Panasyuk, M. I., Nechaev, O. Y., Benghin, V. V., Petrov, V. M, Volkov, A. N., Lyagushin, V. I., & Nikolaev, I. V. 2012. Results of Monitoring Variations of Absorbed Dose Rate onboard the International Space Station during the Period 2005–2011. *Cosmic Research, 50* (5), 391–396.

Lonn, E., Bosch, J., Yusuf, S., Sheridan, P., Pogue, J., Arnold, J.M., Sleight, P., Probstfield, J., Dagenais, G. R., HOPE & HOPE-TOO Trial Investigators. (2011). Effects of long-term vitamin e supplementation on cardiovascular events and cancer: A randomized controlled trial. *Journal of the American Medical Association, 293*(1), 338-347.

Ludwig, A., Lorenz, M., Grimbo, N., Steinle, F., Meiners, S., Bartsch, C., Stangl, K., Baumann, G., & Stangl, V. (2004). The tea flavonoid epigallocatechin-3-gallate reduces cytokine-induced VCAM-1 expression and monocyte adhesion to endothelial cells. *Biochemical and Biophysical Research Communication, 316,* 659-665.

Lusis, A. J. (2000). Atherosclerosis. *Nature, 407,* 233–241.

Lyons, P. D., & Benveniste, E. N. (1998). Cleavage of membrane associated ICAM-1 from astrocytes: involvement of mettalloprotease. *Glia, 22,*103-112.

Maclellan, M. (1983). Palm oil. *Journal of the American Oil Chemists Society, 60* (2), 320A-325A.

MacNaul, K. L., & Hutchinson, N. I. (1993) Differential expression of iNOS and cNOS mRNA in human vascular smooth muscle cells and endothelial cells under normal and inflammatory conditions. *Biochemical and Biophysical Research Communication, 196,* 1330-1334.

Maiese, K., Chong, Z. Z., Hou, J., & Shang, Y. C. (2010). Oxidative stress: biomarkers and novel therapeutic pathways. *Experimental Gerontology. 45(3),* 217-234.

Manka, D. R, Wiegman, P., Din, S., Sanders, J. M., Green, S. A., Gimple, L.W., Ragosta, M., Powers, E. R., Ley, K., & Sarembock, I. J. (1999). Arterial injury increases expression of inflammatory adhesion molecules in the carotid arteries of apolipoprotein-E-deficient mice. *Journal of Vascular Research, 36*(5), 372-378.

Martinez, M. N., Gonzalez-Abuin, N., Terra, X., Richart, C., Ardevol, A., Pinent, M., & Blay, M. (2012). Omega-3 docosahexaenoic acid and procyanidins inhibit cyclo-oxygenase activity and attenuate NF-κB activation through a p105/p50 regulatory mechanism in macrophage inflammation. *Biochemical Journal, 441*(2), 653-663.

McCarty, M. F. (1999). Interleukin-6 as a central mediator of cardiovascular risk associated with chronic inflammation, smoking, diabetes and visceral obesity: down-regulation with essential fatty acids, ethanol and pentoxifylline. *Med-Hypotheses, 52,* 465-477.

Milestone, D. S., Fukumura, D., Padgett, R. C, O'Donnell, P. E., Davis, V. M., Benavidez, O. J., Monsky, W. L., Melder, R. J., Jain, R. K., Gimbrone, M. A. Jr. (1998). Mice lacking E-selectin show normal numbers of rolling leukocytes but reduced leukocyte stable arrest on cytokine-activated microvascular endothelium. *Microcirculation, 5,* 153-171.

Miller, E. R., Barriuso, R. P., Dalal, D., Riemersma, R. A., Appel, L. J., & Guallar, E. (2005). Meta-analysis: High-dosage vitamin E supplementation May Increase All-Cause Mortality. *Annals of Internal Medicine, 142,* 37-46.

Miller, E. S., Koebel D.A., & Sonnenfeld G. (1995). Influence of spaceflight on the production of interleukin-3 and interleukin-6 by rat spleen and thymus cells. *Journal of Applied Physiology, 78,* 810–13.

Mills, P. J., Perez, C. J., Adler, K. A., & Ziegler, M. G. (2002). The effects of space-flight on adrenergic receptors and agonists and cell adhesion molecule expression. *Journal of Neuroimmunology, 132,* 173-9.

Miyazawa, T., Shibata, A., Nakagawa, K., & Tsuzuki, T. (2008). Anti-angiogenic function of tocotrienol. *Asian Pacific Journal of Clinical Nutrition, 17* (Suppl 1), 253-256.

Monaco C., Andreakos, E., Kiriakidis, S., Mauri, C., Bicknell, C., Foxwell, B., Cheshire, N., Paleolog, E., & Feldmann, M. (2004). Canonical pathway of nuclear factor B activation selectively regulates proinflammatory and prothrombotic responses in human atherosclerosis. *Proceedings of the National Academy of Sciences, 101*(15), 5634-5639.

Monici, M., Marziliano, N., Basile V., Pezzatini, S., Romano, G., Conti, A., & Morbidelli, L. (2006). Hypergravity affects morphology and function in microvascular endothelial cells, *Microgravity Science and Technology, 17,* 3-4.

Morbidelli, L., Monici, M., Marziliano N., Cogoli A., Fusi F., Waltenberger J., & Ziche M. (2005). Simulated hypogravity impairs the angiogenic response of endothelium by up-regulating apoptotic signals. *Biochemical and Biophysical Research Communication, 334,* 491-499.

Mosmann, T. (1983). Rapid colorimetric assay for cellular growth and survival: application to proliferation and cytotoxicity assays. *Journal of Immunological Methods, 65*(1-2), 55-63.

Muid, S., Ali. A. M., Yusoff, K., & Nawawi H. (2013). Optimal antioxidant activity with moderate concentrations of tocotrienol in *In Vitro* Assays. *International Food Research Journal, 20*(2), 687-694.

Muid, S., Froemming, G.R.A., Manaf, A., Muszaphar, S., Yusoff, K., & Nawawi, H. (2010). Changes in protein and gene expession of adhesion molecules and cytokines of endothelial cells immediately following short-term spaceflight travel. *Gravitational and Space Biology, 23*(2), S1-11.

Mukherjee, S., & Mitra, A. (2009). Health Effects of Palm Oil. *J Hum Ecol, 26*(3), 197-203.

Munoz-Chapuli, R., Carmona, R., Guadix, J. A., Macias, D., & Perez-Pomares J. M. (2005). The origin of the endothelial cells: an evo-devo approach for the invertebrate/vertebrate transition of the circulatory system. *Evolution & Development, 7* (4), 351-358.

Mustad, V. A., Smith, C. A., Ruey, P. P., Edens, N. K., & Michelle, S. J. (2002). Supplementation with 3 compositionally different tocotrienol supplements does not improve cardiovascular disease risk factors in men and women with hypercholesterolemia. *American Journal of Clinical Nutrition, 76,* 1237-1243.

Naito, Y., Shimozawa, M., Kuroda, M., Nakabe, N., Manabe, H., Katada, K., Kokura, S., Ichikawa, H., Yoshida, N., Noguchi, N., & Yoshikawa, T. (2005). Tocotrienols reduce 25-hydroxycholesterol-induced monocyte-endothelial cell interaction by inhibiting the surface expression of adhesion molecules. *Atherosclerosis, 180,* 19-25.

Naka, T., Nishimoto, N., & Kishimoto, T. (2002). The paradigm of IL-6: from basic science to medicine. *Arthritis Research, 4* (suppl 3), S233-S242.

Nakagawa, K., Shibata, A., Yamashita, S., Tsuzuki, T., Kariya, J., Oikawa, S., Miyazawa, T. (2007). *In vivo* angiogenesis is suppressed by unsaturated vitamin E, tocotrienol. *Journal of Nutrition, 137* (8), 1938-1943.

Nawawi, H, Osman, N. S., Annuar, R., Khalid B. A., & Yusoff, K. (2003). Soluble intercellular adhesion molecule-1 and interleukin-6 levels reflect endothelial dysfunction in patients with primary hypercholesterolemia treated with atorvastatin. *Atherosclerosis, 169,* 283-291.

Nawawi, H., Nor, I. M., Noor, I. M., Karim, N. A, Arshad, F., Khan, R., & Yusoff, K. (2002). Current status of coronary risk factors in rural Malays in Malaysia. *J Cardiovascular Risk, 9*(1), 17-23.

Nesaretnam, K., & Meganathan, P. (2011). Tocotrienols: inflammation and cancer. *Annals of the New York Academy Of Sciences, 1229,* 18-22.

Ng, L. T., & Ko, H. J. (2012). Comparative effects of tocotrienol-rich fraction, a-tocopherol and a-tocopherylacetate on inflammatory mediators and nuclear factor kappa B expression in mouse peritoneal macrophages. *Food Chemistry, 134,* 920–925.

Nishida, K., Harrison, D. G., Navas, J. P., Fisher, A. A., Dockery, S. P., Uematsu, M., Nerem, R. M., Alexander, R. W., & Murphy, T. J. (1992). Molecular cloning and characterization of the constitutive bovine aortic endothelial cell nitric oxide synthase. *Journal of Clinical Investigation, 90,* 2092–2096.

Noguchi, N., Hanyu, R., Nonaka, A., Okimoto, Y., & Kodama, T. (2003). Inhibition of THP-1 cell adhesion to endothelial cells by alpha-tocopherol and alphatocotrienol is dependent on intracellular concentration of the antioxidants. *Free Radical Biology and Medicine, 34,* 1614-1620.

Onat, D., **Brillon**, D., **Colombo**, P. C., **Schmidt**, A. M. (2011). Human Vascular Endothelial Cells: A Model System for Studying Vascular Inflammation in Diabetes and Atherosclerosis. ***Current Diabetes Report, 11***(3), **193–202.**

Orange, J. S., Levy, O., & Geha, R. S. (2005). Human disease resulting from gene mutations that interfere appropriate nuclear factor kappa B activation. *Immunological Reviews, 203,* 21-37.

Orekhov, A. N., Sobenin, I. A., Melnichenko, A. A, Myasoedova, V. A & Bobryshev, Y. V. (2013). Use of Natural Products for Direct Anti-Atherosclerotic Therapy, Current Trends in Atherogenesis, Prof. Rita Rezzani (Ed.), ISBN: 978-953-51-1011-8, InTech, DOI: 10.5772/52967.

Orekhov, A. N., & Tertov, V. V. (1997). *In vitro* effect of garlic powder extract on lipid content in normal and atherosclerotic human aortic cells. *Lipids, 32*(10), 1055-60.

Osiecki, H. (2004). The role of chronic inflammation in cardiovascular disease and its regulation by nutrients. *Alternative Medicine Review, 9* (1), 32-53.

Packard, R. R., & Libby, P. (2008). Inflammation in atherosclerosis: from vascular biology to biomarker discovery and risk prediction. *Clinical Chemistry,* 54 (1), 24-38.

Palozza, P., Verdecchia, S., Avanzi, L., Vertuani, S., Serini, S., Iannone, A., & Manfredini, S. (2006). Comparative antioxidant activity of tocotrienols and the novel chromanyl-polyisoprenyl molecule FeAox-6 in isolated membranes and intact cells. *Molecular and Cellular Biochemistry, 287,* 21-32.

Pamukcu, B., Lip, G. Y. H., & Shantsila, E. (2011). The nuclear factor kappa B pathway in atherosclerosis: A potential therapeutic target for atherothrombotic vascular disease. *Thrombosis Research, 128,* 117-123.

Panes, J., Perry, M. A., Anderson, D. C., Manning, A., Leone, B., Cepinskas, G., Rosenbloom, C. L., Miyasaka, M., Kvietys, P. R., & Granger, D. N. (1995). Regional differences in constitutive and induced ICAM-1 expression *in vivo. American Journal of Physiol*ogy, *269,* H1955-H1964.

Paoletti, R., Gotto, A. M., & Hajjar, D. P. (2004). Inflammation in Atherosclerosis and Implications for Therapy. *Circulation, 109* (Suppl III), III-20-III-26.

Paulsen, K., Thiel, C., Timma, J., Schmidt, P. M., Huber, K., Tauber, S., Hemmersbachd, R., Seibtd, D., Krolle, H., Grotef, K. H., & Zippg, F. (2010). Microgravity-induced alterations in signal transduction in cells of the immune system. *Acta Astronautica, 67,* 1116-1125.

Pearson, J. D. (2000). Normal endothelial cell function. *Lupus, 9* (3), 183-188.

Pendyala, L.K., Yin, X., Li, J., Chen, J. P., Chronos, N., & Hou, D. (2009). The First-Generation Drug-Eluting Stents and Coronary Endothelial Dysfunction. *J Am Coll Cardiol Intv 2*(12), 1169-1177.

Peng, H.B., Libby, P., & Liao, J.K. (1995). Induction and stabilization of IκBα by nitric oxide mediates inhibition of NFκB. *Journal of Biological Chemistry, 270,* 14214-14219.

Pietsch, J., Bauer, J., Egli, M., Infanger, M., Wise, P., Ulbrich, C., & Grimm, D. (2011). The Effects of Weightlessness on the Human Organism and Mammalian Cells. *Current Molecular Medicine 2011, 11,* 350-364.

Pigott, R., Dillon, L. P., Hemingway, I. H., & Gearing, A.J. (1992). Soluble forms of e-selectin, ICAM-1 and VCAM-1 are present in the supernatant of cytokine activated cultured endothelial cells. *Biochem Biophys Res Commun, 187,* 584-589.

Ping, Y. L., &. Reid, M. B. (2001). Effects of tumour necrosis factor-α on skeletal muscle metabolism. *Current Opinion of Rheumatolology, 13,* 483-487.

Pober, J. S. (1998). Activation and injury of endothelial cells by cytokines. *Pathol Biol, 46,*159-163.

Pober, J. S., & Cotran, R. S. (1990). The role of endothelial cells in inflammation. *Transplantation 50,* 537–44.

Porcel, M. R., Lerman, L. O., Holmes Jr., D. R., Richardson, D., Napolic, C., & Lerman, A. (2002). Chronic antioxidant supplementation attenuates nuclear factor-kB activation and preserves endothelial function in hypercholesterolemic pigs. *Cardiovascular Research, 53,* 1010-1018.

Poredos, P. (2011). Markers of preclinical atherosclerosis and their clinical relevance. *The Open Atherosclerosis & Thrombosis Journal, 4,* 1-10.

Pradhan, S., & Sumpio, B. (2004). Molecular and biological effects of hemodynamics on vascular cells. *Frontiers in Bioscience, 9,* 3276-3285.

Qureshi A. A, Reis J. C., Papasian C. J., Morrison, D. C., & Qureshi, N. (2010). Tocotrienols inhibit lipopolysaccharide-induced pro-inflammatory cytokines in macrophages of female mice. *Lipids in Health and Disease, 9*(143), 1-15.

Qureshi, A. A., Burger, D. M., Peterson, C., & Elson, E., (1986). The structure of an inhibitor of cholesterol biosynthesis isolated from barley. *Journal of Biological Chemistry,* 261 (23), 10544-10550.

Qureshi, A. A., Pearce, C., Nor, R. M. Gapor, A., Peterson, D. M., & Elson, C. E. (1996). Dietary d-tocopherol attenuates the impact of d-tocotrienol on hepatic 3-hydroxy-3- methylglutaryl coenzyme A reductase activity in chickens. *Journal of Nutrition, 126,* 389-394.

Qureshi, A. A., Reis, J. C., Qureshi, N., Papasian, C. J., Morrison, D. C., & Schaefer, D. M. (2011). δ-Tocotrienol and quercetin reduce serum levels of nitric oxide and lipid parameters in female chickens. *Lipids in Health and Disease 10*(39), 1-22.

Qureshi, A. A., Sami, S. A., Salser, W. A., & Khan, F. A. (2002). Dose-dependent suppression of serum cholesterol by tocotrienol rich fraction (TRF25) of rice bran in hypercholesterolemic humans. *Atherosclerosis, 161,* 318-329.

Rao, R. M., Yang, L., Cardena, G. G., & Luscinskas F. W. (2007). Endothelial-Dependent Mechanisms of Leukocyte Recruitment to the Vascular Wall. *Circulation Res*earch, *101*, 234.

Reyes, C., Freeman-Perez, S. & Fritsch-Yelle, J. (1999). Orthostatic intolerance following short and long duration spaceflight. *FASEB Journal, 13*, A1048.

Ridker, P. M., Hennekens, C. H., Buring, J. E., & Rifai, N. (2000). C-reactive protein and other markers of inflammation in the prediction of cardiovascular disease in women. *New England Journal of Medicine, 342,* 836-843.

Ridker, P. M., Hennekens, C. H., Johnson, R. B., Stampfer, M. J., & Allen, J. (1998). Plasma concentration of soluble intercellular adhesion molecule-1 and risks of future myocardial infarction in apparently healthy women. *Lancet, 351,* 88-92.

Rietveld, A. & Wiseman, S. (2003). Antioxidant Effects of Tea: Evidence from Human Clinical Trials. *Journal of Nutrition, 133*(10), 3285S-3292S.

Rimm, E. B., Stampfer, M. J., & Ascherio, A. (1993). Vitamin E consumption and the risk of coronary heart disease in men. *New England Journal of Medicine, 328,* 1450-1456.

Rohde, L.E., Lee, R., Rivero, J., Jamacochian, M., Arroyo, L., Briggs W., Rifai N., Libby, P., Creager, M. A., & Ridker, P. M. (1998). Circulating vascular cell adhesion molecule-1 correlates with extent of human atherosclerosis in contrast to circulating intercellular adhesion molecule-1, E-selectin, P-selectin and thrombomodulin. *Arteriosclerosis, Thrombosis & Vascular Biology, 18,* 1765-70.

Roldan, V., Marin, F., Lip, G. Y., & Blann, A. D. (2003). Soluble e-selectine in cardiovascular disease and its risk factors, a review of the literature. *Journal of Thrombosis & Haemostasis, 90,* 1007-1020.

Romanov, Y. A., Buravkova, L. B, Rikova, M. P., Antropova, E. N., Savchenko, N. N., & Kabaeva, N. V. (2001). Expression of cell adhesion molecules and lymphocyte-endothelium interaction under simulated hypogravity *in vitro*. *Journal of Gravitational Physiology, 8*(1), 5-8.

Ross, R., (1999). Atherosclerosis: an inflammatory disease. *New England Journal of Medicine, 340,* 115-126.

Rowe, W. J. (1997). Interplanetary travel and permanent injury to normal heart. *Acta Astronautica, 40,* 719-22.

Rowe, W. J. (1998). The Apollo 15 space syndrome. *Circulation, 97,* 119-20.

Rowe, W.J. (2004). The case for a subcutaneous magnesium product and delivery device for space missions. *Journal of American College of Nutrition, 23*(5), 525S-528S.

Roy, J., Audette, M., & Tremblay, M. J. (2001). Intercellular adhesion molecules-1 (ICAM-1) gene expression in human T cells is regulated by phosphotyrosyl phosphatase activity: involvement of NFκB, Ets and palindromic interferon-responsive element binding sites. *Journal of Biological Chemistry, 276,* 14553-14561.

Rucci, N., Rufo, A., Alamanou M., & Teti A. (2007). Modeled microgravity stimulates osteoclastogenesis and bone resorption by increasing osteoblast RANKL/OPG ratio. *Journal of Cellular Biochemistry,100,* 464–473.

Sadeghi, M. M., Collinge, M., Pardi, R., & Bender, J. R. (2000). Simvastatin modulates cytokine-mediated endothelial cell adhesion molecule induction: Involvement of an inhibitory G protein. *Journal of Immunology, 165,* 2712-2718.

Sata, M., & Fukuda, D. (2011). Chronic inflammation and atherosclerosis: A critical role for renin angiotensin system that is activated by lifestyle-related diseases. *Inflammation and Regeneration, 31* (3), 245-255.

Saura, M., Zaragoza, C., Bao, C., Herranz, B., Puyol, M. R., & Lowenstein, C. J. (2006). STAT-3 Mediates Interleukin-6 Inhibition of Human Endothelial Nitric-oxide Synthase Expression. *The Journal of Biological Chemistry, 281*(40), 30057–30062.

Schuringa, J. J., Dekker, L. V., Vellenga, E., & Kruijer, W. (2001). Sequential activation of Rac-1, SEK-1/MKK-4 and protein kinase C delta is required for IL-6 induced STAT-3 Ser-727 phosphorylation and transactivation. *Journal of Biological Chemistry, 276,* 27709-27715.

Scrivo, R., Vasile, M., Bartosiewicz, I., & Valesini, G. (2011). Inflammation as "common soil" of the multifactorial diseases. *Autoimmunity Reviews, 10,* 139-374.

Seino, Y., Ikeda, U., Ikeda, M., Yamamoto, K., Misawa, Y., Hasegawa, T., Kano, S., & Shimada, K. (1994). Interleukin-6 gene transcripts are expressed in human atherosclerotics lesions. *Cytokine, 6,* 87-91.

Semov, A., Semova, N., Lacelle, C., Marcotte, R., Petroulakis, E., Proestou, G., & Wang, E. (2002). Alterations in TNF- α and IL-related gene expression in space-flown WI38 human fibroblast. *FASEB Journal, 1096* (10), 899-901.

Sen, C. K., Khanna, S., & Roy, S. (2006). Tocotrienols: Vitamin E beyond tocopherols. *Life Sciences, 78,* 2088-2098.

Sen, C. K., Khanna, S, Rink, C., & Roy, S. (2007). Tocotrienols: the emerging face of natural vitamin E. *Vitamins and Hormones, 76,* 203-61.

Serbinova, E., Kagan, V., Han, D., & Packer, L. (1991). Free recycling and intramembrane mobility in antioxidant properties of α-tocopherol and α–tocotrienol. *Free Radical Biology & Medicine,10,* 263-275.

Setiadi D. H., Chass, G. A., Torday, L. L., Varro, A., & Papp, J. C. (2002). Conformational analysis and stereochemistry of tetralin, chroman, thiochroman and selenochroman. *Journal of Molecular Structure 594,* 161-172.

Sharma, C. S., Sarkar S., Periyakaruppan A., Ravichandran P., Sadanandan B., Ramesh, V., et al. (2008). Simulated microgravity activates apoptosis and NF-κB in mice testis. *Molecular and Cellular Biochemistry, 313* (1-2), 71-78.

Shaul, P. W. (2003). Endothelial nitric oxide synthase, caveolae and the development of atherosclerosis. *Journal of Physiology, 547* (1), 21-33.

Sinensky, M., & Lutz, R. (1992). The prenylation of proteins. *Bio Essays, 14,* 25-31.

Soskic S. S., Dobutovi B. D., Sudar , E. M., Obradovi, M. M., Nikoli, D. M., Djordjevic J. D., Radak, D. J., Mikhailidis, D. P., & Isenović, E. R. (2011). Regulation of Inducible Nitric Oxide Synthase (iNOS) and its Potential Role in Insulin Resistance, Diabetes and Heart Failure. *The Open Cardiovascular Medicine Journal, 5*, 153-163.

Spiecker, M., Peng, H. B., & Liao, J. K. (1997). Inhibition of endothelial vascular cell adhesion molecule-1 expression by nitric oxide involves in the induction and nuclear translocation of IκBα. *Journal of Biological Chemistry, 272*, 30969-30974.

Stamenovic, D., Mijailovich, S. M. I., Norrelykke I. M. T., Chen, J., & Wang, N. (2002). Cell prestress. II. Contribution of microtubules. *American Journal of Physiology- Cell Physiology, 282*, C617-C624.

Stein, T. P., & Schluter, M. D. (1994). Excretion of IL-6 by astronauts during spaceflight. *American Journal of Physiology, 266,* E448-52.

Steinberg, D. (2006). An interpretive history of the cholesterol controversy, part V: The discovery of the statins and the end of the controversy. *Journal of Lipid Research,* 1339-1351.

Sultan, S., Gosling, M., Nagase, H., & Powell, J.T. (2004). Shear stress–induced shedding of soluble intercellular adhesion molecule-1 from saphenous vein endothelium. *FEBS Letter, 564*, 161-165.

Sumpio, B. E., Riley, J. T., & Dardik A. (2002). Cells in focus: endothelial cell. *The International Journal of Biochemistry & Cell Biology, 34,* 1508-1512.

Suzuki, T., Miyazawa, T., Fujimoto, K., Otsuka, M., & Tsutsumi, M. (1993). Age-related accumulation of phosphatidylcholine hydroperoxide in cultured human diploid cells and its prevention by α-tocopherol. *Lipids*, 775-778.

Swerdlow, D. I. (2012). The interleukin-6 receptor as a target for prevention of coronary heart disease: a mendelian randomisation analysis. *Lancet, 379*, 1214-1224.

Szmitko, P. E., Wang, C. H., Weisel, R. D., de Almeida, J.R., Anderson, T. J., & Verma S. (2003). New markers of inflammation and endothelial cell activation: Part I. *Circulation, 108,*1917-1923.

Talwar, S., Nandakumar K., Nayak, P. G., Bansal, P., Mudgal, J., Mor V., et al. (2011). Anti-inflammatory activity of Terminalia Paniculata Bark extract against acute and chronic inflammation in rats. *Journal of Ethnopharmacology, 134*, 323-328.

Tan B . 2010. Tocotrienols: the New Vitamin E,. Spacedocnet, www. Spacedoc.net.

Tan, B. (2005). Appropriate Spectrum Vitamin E and New Perspectives on Desmethyl Tocopherols and Tocotrienols. *The Journal of the American Neutricutical Association, 8*(1), 1-15.

Tan, S. W., Ramasamy, R., Abdullah, M., & Vidyadaran, S. (2011). Inhibitory effects of palm a-, c- and d-tocotrienol on lipopolysaccharide-induced nitric oxide production in BV2 microglia. *Cellular Immunology 271*, 205-209.

Tardif, J C. (2006). Prevention challenges: The era of atherosclerosis regression. *Canadian Journal of Cardiology, 22*(Suppl C), 27C-30C.

Theriault, A., Chao, J. T., & Gapor, A. (2002) Tocotrienol is the most effective vitamin E for reducing endothelial expression of adhesion molecules and adhesion to monocytes. *Atherosclerosis, 160,* 21-30.

Theriault, A., Chao, J. T., Wang, Q., Gapor, A., & Adeli, K. (1999). Tocotrienol: A Review of its Therapeutic Potential. *Clinical Biochemistry, 32*(5), 309-319.

Thusen, J. H. V. D., Kuiper, J., Van Berkel, T. G. C., & Biessen, E. A. L. (2003). Interleukins in atherosclerosis: Molecular pathways and therapeutic potential. *Pharmacological Reviews, 55* (1): 133-166.

Tian, J., Pecaut, M. J., Slater, J. M., & Gridley, D. S. (2010). Spaceflight Modulates Expression of Extracellular Matrix, Adhesion and Profibrotic Molecules in Mouse Lung. *Journal of Applied Physiology,* 108, 162-171.

Tracey, K. J., & Cerami, A. (1990). Metabolic responses to cachectin/TNF. A brief review. *Annals of New York Academy of Sciences, 587*, 325-331.

Tsakadze, N. L., Zhoa, Z., & D' Souza, S. E. (2002). Interactions of intercellular adhesion molecule-1 with fibrinogen. *Trends in Cardiovascular Medicine, 12,* 101-108.

Valencia, H. A., & Mills, J. M. C. (2006). VCAM-1 Signals Activate Endothelial Cell Protein Kinase C via Oxidation1. *The Journal of Immunology, 177,* 6379–6387.

Vallance, P., & Chan, N. (2001). Endothelial function and nitric oxide: clinical relevance. *Heart, 85,* 342-350.

Vasanthi, H. R., Parameswari, R. P., & Das, D. K. (2012). Multifaceted role of tocotrienols in cardioprotection supports their structure: function relation. *Genes Nutrition, 7(1),* 19-28.

Vaziri, N. D., Ding. Y., Sangha, D. S., & Purdy, R. E. (2000). Upregulation of NOS by simulated microgravity, potential cause of arthostatic intolerance. *Journal of Applied Physiology, 89,* 338-344.

Versari, S., Villa A., Bradamante S., & Maier J. A. M. (2007). Alterations of the actin cytoskeleton and increased nitric oxide synthesis are common features in human primary endothelial cell response to changes in gravity. *Biochimica et Biophysica Acta, 1773*(11), 1645-1652.

Vestweber, D., & Blanks, J. E. (1999). Mechanisms that regulate the function of the selectines and their ligands. *Physiological Reviews, 79,* 181-213.

Villa, A., Versari, S., Maier, J. A. M., & Bradamante, S. (2005). Cell behavior in simulated microgravity: A Comparison of results obtained with RWV and RPM. *Gravitational and Space Biology, 18* (2), 89-90.

Wallen, N. H., Held, C., Rehnqivst, N., & Hjemdahl, P. (1999). Elevated serum intercellular adhesion molecule-1 and vascular cell adhesion molecule -1 among patients with stable angina pectoris who suffer cardiovascular death or non-fatal myocardial infarction. *European Heart Journal, 20,* 1039-1043.

Weber, C., Erl, W., Weber, K. S. C., & Weber, P. C. (1997). HMG-CoA reductase inhibitors decrease CD11b expression and CD11b-dependent adhesion of monocytes to endothelium and reduce increased adhesiveness of monocytes isolated from hypercholesterolemic patients. *Journal of American College of Cardiology, 30,* 1212-1217.

White, R. J., & Averner, M. (2001). Humans in space. *Nature, 409,* 1115-1118.

Willerson, J. T., & Ridker, P. M. (2004). Inflammation as a cardiovascular risk factor. *Circulation, 109* (Suppl II), II-2-II-10.

Winther, M.P.J., Kanters, E., Kraal, G., & Hofker, M.H. (2005). Nuclear Factor κB signaling in atherogenesis. *Arteriosclerosis, Thrombosis & Vascular Biology, 25*, 904-914.

Wise, K. C., Manna, S. K., Yamauchi, K., Ramesh, V., Ramesh G. T., Thomas, R. L., Sarkar, S., Kulkarni. A. D., Pellis, N. R, & Ramesh, G. T. (2005). Activation of nuclear transcription factor-kappaB in mouse brain induced by a simulated microgravity environment. *In Vitro Cellular & Developmental Biology, 41* (3-4), 118-23.

Wood, S. C., Bushar, G., & Tesfamariam, B. (2006). Inhibition of mammalian target of rapamycin modulates expression of adhesion molecules in endothelial cells. *Toxicology Letter, 165,* 242-249.

Wu, S. J., Liu, P. L., & Lean-Teik, N. (2008). Tocotrienol-rich fraction of palm oil exhibits anti-inflammatory property by suppressing the expression of inflammatory mediators in human monocytic cells. *Molecular Nutrition & Food Research, 52,*921-929.

Wung, B. S., Ni, C. W., & Wang, D. L. (2005). ICAM-1 induction by TNF-α and IL-6 is mediated by distinct pathways via Rac in endothelial cells. *Journal of Biomedical Sciences, 12* (1), 91-101.

Yam, M. L., Abdul Hafid, S. R., Cheng, H. M., & Nesaretnam, K. (2009) Tocotrienols suppress proinflammatory markers and cyclooxygenase- 2 expression in RAW264.7 macrophages. *Lipids, 44,* 787–797.

Yamashita, H., Shimada, K., Seki, E., Mokuna, H., & Daida, H. (2003). Concentrations of interleukins, interferon and C-reactive protein in stable and unstable angina pectoris. *American Journal of Cardiology, 91,* 133-136.

Yang, X. P., Irani, K., Mattagajasingh, S., DiPaula, A., Khanday, F., Ozaki M., Fox-Talbot, K., Baldwin, W. M., & Becker, L. C. (2005). Signal transducer and activator of transcription 3α and specificity protein 1 interact to upregulate intercellular adhesion molecule-1 in ischemic-reperfused myocardium and vascular endothelium. *Arteriosclerosis Thrombosis & Vascular Biology, 25,*1395-1400.

Yoshida, Y., Niki, E., & Noguchi, N. (2003). Comparative Study on the action of tocopherols and tocotrienols as an antioxidant: chemical and physical effects. *Chemistry and Physics of Lipids, 123,* 63-75.

Yu, Y., Moulton, K. S., Khan, M. K., Vineberg, S., Boye, E., Davis, V. M. O'Donnellm P. E., Bischoff, J., Milstone, D. S. (2004). E-selectin is required for the antiangiogenic activity of endostatin. *Proceedings of the National Academy of Sciences of The United States of America, 101*(21), 8005-8010.

Yudkin, J. S., Kumari, M., Humphries, S. E., & Mohamed-Ali, V. (2000). Inflammation, obesity, stress and coronary heart disease: is Interleukin 6 the link? *Atherosclerosis, 148,* 209-214.

Zhang, H., Park, Y., Wu, J., Chen, X. P., Lee, S., Yang, J., Dellsperger, K. C., & Zhang, C. (2009). Role of TNF-α in vascular dysfunction. *Clinical Science, 116,* 219-230.

Zhang, H., & Zhang, C. (2011). Vasoprotection by Dietary Supplements and Exercise: Role of TNF-α Signaling. *Experimental Diabetes Research, 2012,* 1-6.

Zhang, J., DeFelice, A. F., Hanig, J. P., & Colatsky, T. 2010. Biomarkers of endothelial cell activation serve as potential surrogate markers for drug-induced vascular injury. *Toxicology Pathology, 38,* 856-871.

Zhang, J., Patel, J. M., Li, Y. D., & Block, E. R. (1997). Proinflammatory cytokines downregulate gene expression and activity of constitutive nitric oxide synthase in porcine pulmonary artery endothelial cells. *Research Communications in Molecular Pathology & Pharmacology, 96,* 71-87.

Zhang, R., Ran, H. H., Gao, Y. L., Ma, J., Huang, Y., Bai Y. G., & Lin, L. J. (2010). Differential vascular cell adhesion molecule-1 expression and superoxide production in stimulated microgravity rat vasculature. *EXCLI Journal, 9,* 195-204.

Zhang, R., Jia G., Bao J., Zhang Y., Bai Y., Lin, L., Tang, H., & Ma, J. (2008). Increased Vascular Cell Adhesion Molecule–1 Was Associated with Impaired Endothelium–Dependent Relaxation of Cerebral and Carotid Arteries in Simulated Microgravity Rats. *The Journal of Physiological Sciences, 58* (1), 67-73.

Zhang, X., Lynch, A. L., Davis, B. R., Ford, C. E., Boerwinkle, E., Eckfeldt, J. H., Leiendecker-Foster, C., & Arnett, D. K. (2012). Pharmacogenetic Association of NOS3 Variants with Cardiovascular Disease in Patients with Hypertension: The GenHAT Study. *Plos One, 7* (3), e34217.

Zhang, Y., Sang, C., Paulsen, K., Arenz, A., Zhao, Z., Jia, X., Ullrich, O., & Zhuang, F. (2010). ICAM-1 expression and organization in human endothelial cells is sensitive to gravity. *Acta Astronautica, 67,* 1073-1080.

ABOUT THE AUTHOR

Professor Hapizah Mohd Nawawi; MD (UKM), DCP (London), MSc (London), MRCPath (UK), FRCPath (UK), FAMM (Mal), is a Professor and Senior Consultant in Chemical Pathology and Metabolic Medicine at the Faculty of Medicine, Universiti Teknologi MARA (UiTM), Malaysia; and Director of I-PPerForM, one of the University Centres of Research Excellence, with niches areas in Atherosclerosis and Familial Hypercholesterolaemia (FH). She pioneered and is the Consultant Physician-in-charge of the Specialist Lipids and Coronary Risk Prevention Clinics at the UiTM Teaching Hospital.

Her clinical and research interest is in the field of lipidology, dyslipidaemias including molecular basis of FH, atherosclerosis, coronary risk factors and novel biomarkers, anti-oxidants and coronary artery disease prevention. She has attracted multiple national and international competitive research grants and pharmaceutical industrial support (7.6 million MYR over 20 years). She had headed several competitive research grants in the field of FH, lipidology and atherosclerosis, ranging from basic fundamental science to in-vivo animal and human studies, clinical trials and epidemiological studies. She had led several FH projects, and is currently leading a national research programme on FH, and has pioneered the Malaysian National FH Registry and Genetic Testing Laboratory.

Her key publications are in areas of FH, atherosclerosis and novel biomarkers of atherogenesis. To date, she has about 140 publications including 135 full papers in international and national journals/indexed proceedings and 5 books/chapters in books; 486 abstracts in indexed journals and proceedings, with over 2587/ 853 citations and h-index of 17/13 (GS and Scopus respectively). Currently, she is supervising 4 postgraduate students, in addition to two post-Docs. To date she has graduated a total of 56 postgraduates, including 25 PhDs/PhD equivalents.

Made in United States
North Haven, CT
24 December 2023

46540304R00072